Therapeutic Exercises Using Foam Rollers

Caroline Corning Creager

Executive Physical Therapy, Inc.

Berthoud, Colorado

Library of Congress Card Catalog Number: 96-086360
Creager, Caroline Corning
        Therapeutic Exercises Using Foam Rollers.
        Creager, Caroline Corning - 1st edition, 8th printing.

            Executive Physical Therapy, Inc.
            P.O. Box 1319
            Berthoud, CO 80513 USA
            (970) 532-2533 or 1-800-530-6878
            email: Caroline_Creager@unforgettable.com
            web site: www.CarolineCreager.com

The author has made every effort to assure that the information in this book is accurate and current at the time of printing. The publisher and author take no responsibility for the use of the material in this book and cannot be held responsible for any typographical or other errors found. Please consult your physician before initiating this exercise program. The information in this book is not intended to replace medical advice.

ISBN: 0-9641153-3-6
Library of Congress Card Catalog Number: 96-086360
Printed in the United States of America
First Printing August 1996
Second Printing August 1998
Third Printing October 1999
Fourth Printing April 2001
Fifth Printing November 2002
Sixth Printing June 2004
Seventh Printing January 2006
Eighth Printing October 2008
Ninth Printing June 2012

Book design by Caroline Corning Creager
Composition by Alan Bernhard
Cover design by Paulette Livers Lambert
Photography by Marc Nader
Edited by Caryl Riedel
Hair and Makeup by Cathy Arentz
Drawings by Amy Belg

                    Distributed by:
          Orthopedic Physical Therapy Products
        P.O. Box 47009, Minneapolis, MN 55447, USA
              (612)553-0452 (800)367-7393

About the Author

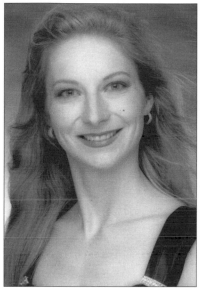

© Marc Nader, 1994

Caroline Corning Creager is an award-winning author and nationally recognized lecturer on the Swiss Ball and Foam Rollers. She received her degree in physical therapy from the University of Montana in 1989. She is the owner of Executive Physical Therapy, Inc., in Berthoud, Colorado, and is a member of the American Physical Therapy Association, the Rocky Mountain Book Publishers Association and the Colorado Independent Publishers Association. Caroline is the author of *Therapeutic Exercises Using the Swiss Ball, The Airobic Ball™ Strengthening Workout,* and *The Airobic Ball™ Stretching Workout.* Her goal is to enhance health care professionals' understanding of how the foam rollers can be used to facilitate individualized clinical, home, and work exercise programs.

Dedication

To my husband, Robert, for adding magic,
mystery, and love into our relationship.

To the students who have participated in my
courses; thank you for sharing new ideas and
techniques with me.

To my co-workers, Jeanne Brexa, Lucy Judson,
and Carole Varga, for the opportunity to share
my exorbitant thoughts, ideas, and experiences.

Acknowledgments

To Brian Hauswirth, P.T., C.F.P., for providing practical experience to the Case Study – One.

To Barbara Headley, M.S., P.T., for contributing her knowledge and expertise of electromyography to the Electromyography Case Study – Three.

To Anne Dawdy, P.T., for contributing information to the Treatment Protocols for Foam Rollers.

To Janet A. Hulme, M.A., P.T., for editing the Breathing chapter and Doug Dewey, P.T., O.C.S., for editing the Treatment Protocols section.

In Memory of Robert Cermely

FOOTSTEPS OF ANGELS

When the hours of Day are numbered,
    And the voices of the Night
Wake the better soul, that slumbered,
    To a holy, calm delight;

Ere the evening lamps are lighted,
    And, like phantoms grim and tall,
Shadows from the fitful firelight
    Dance upon the parlor wall;

Then the forms of the departed
    Enter at the open door;
The beloved, the true-hearted,
    Come to visit me once more;

He, the young and strong, who cherished
    Noble longings for the strife,
By the roadside fell and perished,
    Weary with the march of life!

They, the holy ones and weakly,
    Who the cross of suffering bore,
Folded their pale hands so meekly,
    Spake with us on earth no more!

And with them the Being Beauteous,
    Who unto my youth was given,
More than all things else to love me,
    And is now a saint in heaven.

With a slow and noiseless footstep
    Comes that messenger divine,
Takes the vacant chair beside me,
    Lays her gentle hand in mine.

And she sits and gazes at me
    With those deep and tender eyes,
Like the stars, so still and saint-like,
    Looking downward from the skies.

Uttered not, yet comprehended,
    Is the spirit's voiceless prayer,
Soft rebukes, in blessings ended,
    Breathing from her lips of air.

Oh, though oft depressed and lonely,
    All my fears are laid aside,
If I but remember only
    Such as these have lived and died!

HENRY WADSWORTH LONGFELLOW

Preface

The focus of this book is to improve individualized clinical, work, recreational and home exercise programs by providing illustrated and easy-to-read instructions. This book provides more than 175 illustrated exercise options for the therapist, chiropractor or physician to photocopy for patient use and create a comprehensive foam roller exercise program.

Exercises are categorized by body position on the ball, and are listed by both common and technical names. The PURPOSE of the exercises and the INSTRUCTIONS are written in laymen's terms. Each page provides a SPECIAL PROTOCOLS/NOTES section to allow the therapist to modify the exercise and individualize each patient program.

CASE STUDIES and TREATMENT PROTOCOLS using foam rollers provide the clinician with examples of how to integrate the foam rollers into a treatment regimen. The ELECTRO-MYOGRAPHY STUDY using five of the foam roller exercises from this book is included to help identify the intensity of specific muscles firing during a given exercise.

Proper breathing is such an integral part of any exercise that I included the Breathing chapter. The Breathing chapter provides an introduction to diaphragmatic breathing and can be used with all of the exercises in this book.

After writing and typing this book on my keyboard I decided to include the Computer Fitness Guidelines chapter, to familiarize the clinician with how to arrange and adjust a computer workstation. Foam roller stretching exercises, as in chapter four, can be executed at the workstation as well.

I hope the exercises in this book help to augment each clinician's repertoire of exercises using foam rollers. Furthermore, I encourage each clinician to create new exercises substituting different sized rollers to help facilitate the individual needs of their patients.

CAROLINE CORNING CREAGER, P.T.

Contents

Parallel Developments

". . . there are at least another hundred
people investigating this (the Method) from
another angle. They have the same sort of
insight. When a culture evolves and something is
new, it is impossible that human brains are so
different from one another (even though brains
are different), that important developments do
not occur in ten, a hundred, or even a thousand
places at this moment . . . this generation is a
crucial one. The next generation, or maybe at
the end of this one, what we thought, or what
our parents thought, or what the majority of
people think, will be considered as backwards as
the Middle Ages. There will be an extraordinary
change. There will be a crossing of many
disciplines."

—Moshe Feldenkrais
July 1977

CHAPTER ONE

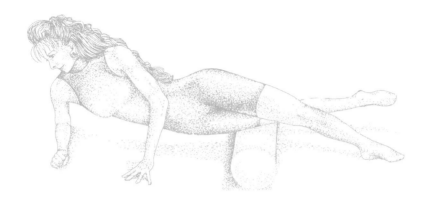

Principles and Concepts of Foam Rollers

Introduction

Foam rollers are cylindrical in shape, lightweight, and vary in length, circumference, and density. The foam roller's design provides sensory motor challenges on two planes and enhances balance reactions, body awareness, muscle reeducation, motor planning, dynamic strengthening, and neural and muscular flexibility.

Foam rollers also add diversification to an exercise regimen by allowing the patient to exercise with the rollers in almost any position: standing, sitting, supine, sidelying, kneeling, quadriped, and prone. For example, a bedridden patient afflicted with Parkinson's disease can utilize the foam rollers in the supine position while in bed to improve strength and endurance, whereas a patient with an anterior cruciate ligament repair may use the roller while standing to promote proprioceptive awareness.

According to Brian Hauswirth, P.T., Certified Feldenkrais Practitioner (C.F.P.) and owner of Integrating Function Physical Therapy, Larkspur, CA: "Foam rollers provide the patient with immediate reinforcement as to how they are progressing with their exercises and a sense of accomplishment when the patient is able to complete the exercises while maintaining balance."

Ilana Parker, P.T., C.F.P., owner of Ilana Physical Therapy, San Francisco, CA, wrote in *Beyond Conventional Exercise*: "Exercises on these surfaces [foam rollers] are simple, economical, and fun."[1]

Furthermore, Elsa Nail, M.S., P.T., Clearwater, FL, states: "Patient compliance is high because foam rollers do not require time and effort to set up or use."[2]

Most foam rollers are comprised of polyethylene. Cross-linked polyethylene is found in running shoes and medical appliances whereas Ethafoam®, made solely of polyethylene, is used for packaging equipment. Foam rollers, commonly used by physical therapists and other health care professionals, are made from Ethafoam® as well.

Another type of roller, not as common nor as readily available as the Ethafoam® roller, is made from polyurethane. Polyurethane constitutes a softer foam roller which provides less stability. However, it may add more comfort when lying prone or supine on the rollers.

Dow Chemical originally began manufacturing foam rounds or rollers as athletic equipment, such as tumbling mats, and as packaging material for items such as automotive parts. In addition, children currently use foam rollers in the swimming pool as floating devices, and health care professionals use them as therapeutic tools in treatment regimens.

Dr. Moshe Feldenkrais (1902–1984), physicist and founder of the Feldenkrais Method, has been credited with being one of the first individuals to begin using rollers as a therapeutic tool.[3, 4] In the late 1950s, Feldenkrais began using wooden rollers to help lessen the frictional component of a moving body part on a plinth and to reduce muscular activity in a static position (i.e., placing a roller under the knees in a supine position)[5]. In 1972, after arriving in the United States to present his work at health institutions and universities, Feldenkrais was introduced to the foam roller. Thereafter he began using the foam rollers in his practice as well.

Osa Jackson Wynn, Ph.D., P.T.; Brian Hainsworth, P.T., C.F.P.; Kent Keyser, M.S., P.T., A.T.C., O.C.S.; Frank Wildman, Ph.D.; Ilana Parker, P.T., C.F.P.; Elsa Nail, M.S., P.T.; David Zemach-Bersin, B.S., C.F.P.; and Mark Reese, Ph.D., C.F.P., have all been influential in the instruction of the foam rollers through the United States.

FOAM ROLLER SIZES

A variety of roller sizes as used in this book are recommended. The following set of foam rollers is recommended for

use with this book (see Figure 1):
 One full roller — 3' by 6"
 One half roller — 3' by 3"
 Two small rollers — 1' by 6"
 Two small half rollers — 1' by 3"

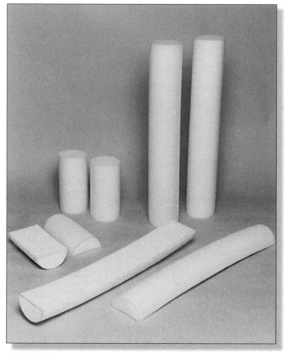

FIGURE 1

Several exercises such as the thoracic and lumbar massage and the standing skier exercise require two or more full rollers.

The cylindrical shape of the full large and small foam rollers yields less contact area on the floor, moves more quickly, and, therefore, challenges balance reactions more than a half roller with its flat surface toward the floor. Standing full foam roller exercises are recommended for the advanced level client.

Half rollers typically provide greater stability thereby making the exercises easier. Half rollers are recommended for prone exercises and may be used in supine positions as well for added comfort. When working with a neurologically involved patient, place the foot on the half roller, flat surface toward foot, instead of rounded surface toward foot. Weight bearing of the feet into the rounded surface of the roller may elicit flexor tone.

Small rollers allow one foot to remain static and the opposite foot to become dynamic as in ballet positions II, IV, and V (pages 109, 110, and 111). Also, by using small rollers, the feet may move in opposite directions as in the quadratus lumborum hip hike exercise (page 195).

After familiarizing yourself with the exercises presented in this book, substitute a different sized roller than the one depicted in an exercise. For example, try using a half roller in the exercise illustrated on page 103, or a half roller for the supine neutral position exercise on page 150.

FOAM ROLLER CARE INSTRUCTIONS

Foam rollers are durable and can hold more than 300 pounds of weight. Moreover, the lightweight Ethafoam® material can be cut easily with a bread knife to change the roller size or shape.

The buoyant nature of the foam rollers makes them excellent floating devices for relaxation exercises, and additional tools for aquatic exercises. The foam rollers, however, are not intended to be used as a life preserver.

In the clinic, cover rollers with towels, sheets or pillowcases or clean rollers with infection control agents, between patients, to prevent cross contamination. At home, clean the foam rollers with soap and water.

PROTOCOLS FOR USING FOAM ROLLERS

INDICATIONS
1. decreased range of motion
2. decreased strength
3. decreased balance reactions
4. decreased coordination
5. decreased endurance
6. decreased proprioception
7. decreased flexibility in myofascial and scar tissue
8. decreased motor planning
9. decreased neural flexibility

PRECAUTIONS
1. muscular fatigue
2. cardiovascular distress
   a. shortness of breath
   b. light-headedness
   c. pallor
   d. nausea
   e. angina
3. adhering to weight restrictions (i.e., non-weight bearing, partial weight bearing, etc.)
4. aggravating degenerative joint disease with mobility exercises
5. following specific injury precautions (i.e., do not exceed 90 degrees of hip flexion with new total hip replacement patients)
6. superseding patient tolerance level
7. recognizing signs of sensory overload
   a. pupil dilation
   b. sweaty palms
   c. changes in respiration rate
   d. flushing or pallor
   e. complaints of dizziness

8. maintaining appropriate supervision and guidance for each patient level
9. using gait belts for all patients
10. keeping foam rollers away from flammable objects

CONTRAINDICATIONS
1. increased pain
2. dizziness/nausea
3. ringing in ears
4. foam roller activities frighten patient
5. full weight-bearing activities on joints with ligamentous laxity
6. any inexperienced foam roller exerciser doing activities without supervision

TREATMENT PROTOCOLS WITH FOAM ROLLERS

The following information is designed to help the clinician become acquainted with the use of the foam roller in a treatment situation. Each individual patient is unique and may vary from the criterion presented below. Please use good judgment and common sense when applying this information to your patients. Use the following information only as a reference and guide to your treatments; observe the patient's signs and symptoms, then carefully and methodically apply your own skills to bring about a positive treatment outcome.[6]

CARPAL TUNNEL SYNDROME
Carpal tunnel syndrome may be the result of one or more of the following: repetitive motion, trauma, pregnancy, collagen disease, etc. The median nerve travels through the carpal tunnel and becomes compressed with inflammation or narrowing of the carpal tunnel itself. Identify any source from the work or home

environment that may be causing the patient to perform the same motions repetitively, and then reduce or eliminate this motion from their routine. Reduce inflammation with appropriate modalities. Instruct patient in soft tissue mobilization and gentle stretching and strengthening exercises.

Wrist Flexor Stretch

PURPOSE: To stretch front side of wrist.

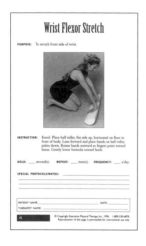

INSTRUCTION: Kneel. Place half roller, flat side up, horizontal on floor in front of body. Lean forward and place hands on half roller, palms down. Rotate hands outward so fingers point toward knees. Gently lower buttocks toward heels.

HOLD: ___ second(s). **REPEAT:** ___ time(s). **FREQUENCY:** ___ x/day.

SPECIAL PROTOCOLS/NOTES: _____

PATIENT NAME: _____ DATE: _____
THERAPIST NAME: _____

42 © Copyright Executive Physical Therapy, Inc., 1996. 1-800-530-6878. Reproduction of this page is permissible for instructional use only.

Wrist Extensor Stretch

PURPOSE: To stretch back side of wrist.

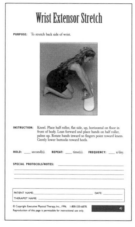

INSTRUCTION: Kneel. Place half roller, flat side up, horizontal on floor in front of body. Lean forward and place hands on half roller, palms up. Rotate hands inward so fingers point toward knees. Gently lower buttocks toward heels.

HOLD: ___ second(s). **REPEAT:** ___ time(s). **FREQUENCY:** ___ x/day.

SPECIAL PROTOCOLS/NOTES: _____

PATIENT NAME: _____ DATE: _____
THERAPIST NAME: _____

© Copyright Executive Physical Therapy, Inc., 1996. 1-800-530-6878. Reproduction of this page is permissible for instructional use only. 43

Prone Tuck

PURPOSE: To increase range of motion in back and knees. To strengthen abdominal, arm, back, and neck muscles.

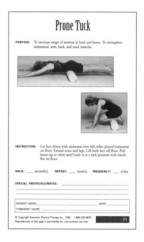

INSTRUCTION: Lie face down with abdomen over full roller placed horizontal on floor. Extend arms and legs. Lift both feet off floor. Pull knees up to chest until body is in a tuck position with hands flat on floor.

HOLD: ___ second(s). **REPEAT:** ___ time(s). **FREQUENCY:** ___ x/day.

SPECIAL PROTOCOLS/NOTES: _____

PATIENT NAME: _____ DATE: _____
THERAPIST NAME: _____

© Copyright Executive Physical Therapy, Inc., 1996. 1-800-530-6878. Reproduction of this page is permissible for instructional use only. 211

Brachioplexus Stretch

PURPOSE: To stretch shoulder and chest muscles.

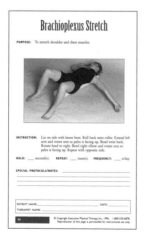

INSTRUCTION: Lie on side with knees bent. Roll back onto roller. Extend left arm and rotate arm so palm is facing up. Bend wrist back. Rotate head to right. Bend right elbow and rotate arm so palm is facing up. Repeat with opposite side.

HOLD: ___ second(s). **REPEAT:** ___ time(s). **FREQUENCY:** ___ x/day.

SPECIAL PROTOCOLS/NOTES: _____

PATIENT NAME: _____ DATE: _____
THERAPIST NAME: _____

44 © Copyright Executive Physical Therapy, Inc., 1996. 1-800-530-6878. Reproduction of this page is permissible for instructional use only.

Shoulder Stretch

PURPOSE: To stretch shoulder muscles.

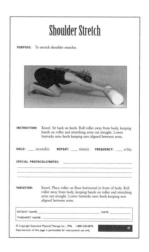

INSTRUCTION: Kneel. Sit back on heels. Roll roller away from body, keeping hands on roller and stretching arms out straight. Lower buttocks onto heels keeping ears aligned between arms.

HOLD: ___ second(s). **REPEAT:** ___ time(s). **FREQUENCY:** ___ x/day.

SPECIAL PROTOCOLS/NOTES: _____

VARIATION: Kneel. Place roller on floor horizontal in front of body. Roll roller away from body, keeping hands on roller and stretching arms out straight. Lower buttocks onto heels keeping ears aligned between arms.

PATIENT NAME: _____ DATE: _____
THERAPIST NAME: _____

© Copyright Executive Physical Therapy, Inc., 1996. 1-800-530-6878. Reproduction of this page is permissible for instructional use only. 45

LATERAL EPICONDYLITIS

Lateral epicondylitis usually affects the dominant arm of adults between the ages of 20 and 50 years old. Inflammation and pain is generally located over the lateral epicondylar region. Reduce inflammation with the appropriate modality. Evaluate and modify the workplace or athletic equipment. Instruct the patient in soft tissue mobilization, and stretching and strengthening exercises for the forearm extensors, especially the extensor carpi radialis brevis and extensor digitoram muscles. These muscles are infamous for contributing to the lateral epicondylitis problem.

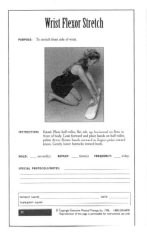

Wrist Flexor Stretch

PURPOSE: To stretch front side of wrist.

INSTRUCTION: Kneel. Place half roller, flat side, up, horizontal on floor in front of body. Lean forward and place hands on half roller, palms down. Rotate hands outward so fingers point toward knees. Gently lower buttocks toward heels.

HOLD: ___ second(s). REPEAT: ___ time(s). FREQUENCY: ___ x/day.

SPECIAL PROTOCOLS/NOTES: _____

PATIENT NAME: _____ DATE: _____
THERAPIST NAME: _____

© Copyright Executive Physical Therapy, Inc., 1996. 1-800-530-6878
Reproduction of this page is permissible for instructional use only

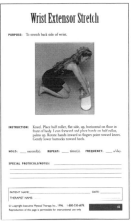

Wrist Extensor Stretch

PURPOSE: To stretch back side of wrist.

INSTRUCTION: Kneel. Place half roller, flat side, up, horizontal on floor in front of body. Lean forward and place hands on half roller, palms up. Rotate hands inward so fingers point toward knees. Gently lower buttocks toward heels.

HOLD: ___ second(s). REPEAT: ___ time(s). FREQUENCY: ___ x/day.

SPECIAL PROTOCOLS/NOTES: _____

PATIENT NAME: _____ DATE: _____
THERAPIST NAME: _____

© Copyright Executive Physical Therapy, Inc., 1996. 1-800-530-6878
Reproduction of this page is permissible for instructional use only

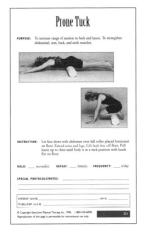

Prone Tuck

PURPOSE: To increase range of motion in back and knees. To strengthen abdominal, arm, back, and neck muscles.

INSTRUCTION: Lie face down with abdomen over full roller placed horizontal on floor. Extend arms and legs. Lift back feet off floor. Pull knees up to chest until body is in a tuck position with hands flat on floor.

HOLD: ___ second(s). REPEAT: ___ time(s). FREQUENCY: ___ x/day.

SPECIAL PROTOCOLS/NOTES: _____

PATIENT NAME: _____ DATE: _____
THERAPIST NAME: _____

© Copyright Executive Physical Therapy, Inc., 1996. 1-800-530-6878
Reproduction of this page is permissible for instructional use only

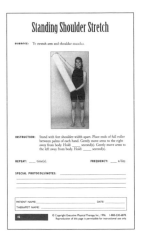

Standing Shoulder Stretch

PURPOSE: To stretch arm and shoulder muscles.

INSTRUCTION: Stand with feet shoulder-width apart. Place ends of full roller between palms of each hand. Gently move arms to the right away from body. Hold ___ second(s). Gently move arms to the left away from body. Hold ___ second(s).

REPEAT: ___ time(s). FREQUENCY: ___ x/day.

SPECIAL PROTOCOLS/NOTES: _____

PATIENT NAME: _____ DATE: _____
THERAPIST NAME: _____

© Copyright Executive Physical Therapy, Inc., 1996. 1-800-530-6878
Reproduction of this page is permissible for instructional use only

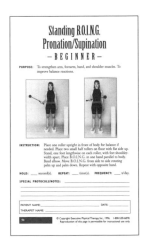

Standing B.O.I.N.G.
Pronation/Supination
– BEGINNER –

PURPOSE: To strengthen arm, forearm, hand, and shoulder muscles. To improve balance reactions.

INSTRUCTION: Place one roller upright in front of body for balance if needed. Place two small half rollers on floor with flat side up. Stand, one foot lengthwise on each roller, with feet shoulder-width apart. Place B.O.I.N.G. in one hand parallel to body. Bend elbow. Move B.O.I.N.G. from side to side rotating palm up and palm down. Repeat with opposite hand.

HOLD: ___ second(s). REPEAT: ___ time(s). FREQUENCY: ___ x/day.

SPECIAL PROTOCOLS/NOTES: _____

PATIENT NAME: _____ DATE: _____
THERAPIST NAME: _____

© Copyright Executive Physical Therapy, Inc., 1996. 1-800-530-6878
Reproduction of this page is permissible for instructional use only

ROTATOR CUFF TEAR

The rotator cuff is made up of four muscles, including the supraspinatus, infraspinatus, teres minor, and subscapularis. The supraspinatus muscle is most commonly ruptured, especially at its insertion. Follow postsurgical precautions and contra-indications. When appropriate progress has been made, graduate the patient from passive to active assistive to active range of motion and strengthening exercises.

Standing Shoulder Stretch

PURPOSE: To stretch arms and shoulder muscles.

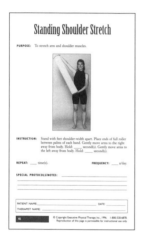

INSTRUCTION: Stand with feet shoulder-width apart. Place ends of full roller between palms of each hand. Gently move arms to the right away from body. Hold ___ second(s). Gently move arms to the left away from body. Hold ___ second(s).

REPEAT: ___ time(s). **FREQUENCY:** ___ x/day.

SPECIAL PROTOCOLS/NOTES: _____

PATIENT NAME: _____ DATE: _____
THERAPIST NAME: _____

© Copyright Executive Physical Therapy, Inc., 1996. 1-800-530-6878.
Reproduction of this page is permissible for instructional use only.

Deltoid Stretch

PURPOSE: To stretch shoulder muscles.

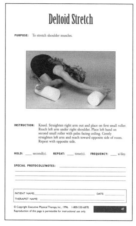

INSTRUCTION: Kneel. Straighten right arm out and place on first small roller. Reach left arm under right shoulder. Place left hand on second small roller with palm facing ceiling. Gently straighten left arm and reach toward opposite side of room. Repeat with opposite side.

HOLD: ___ second(s). **REPEAT:** ___ time(s). **FREQUENCY:** ___ x/day.

SPECIAL PROTOCOLS/NOTES: _____

PATIENT NAME: _____ DATE: _____
THERAPIST NAME: _____

© Copyright Executive Physical Therapy, Inc., 1996. 1-800-530-6878.
Reproduction of this page is permissible for instructional use only.

Standing Resistive Band Shoulder Internal Rotation
– B E G I N N E R –

PURPOSE: To strengthen shoulder muscles.

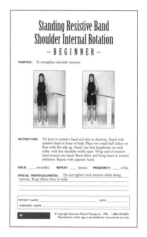

INSTRUCTION: Tie knot in resistive band and shut in doorway. Stand with resistive band in front of body. Place two small half rollers on floor with flat side up. Stand, one foot lengthwise on each roller, with feet shoulder-width apart. Wrap end of resistive band around one hand. Bend elbow and bring hand in toward abdomen. Repeat with opposite hand.

HOLD: ___ second(s). **REPEAT:** ___ time(s). **FREQUENCY:** ___ x/day.

SPECIAL PROTOCOLS/NOTES: Do not tighten neck muscles while doing exercise. Keep elbow close to body.

PATIENT NAME: _____ DATE: _____
THERAPIST NAME: _____

© Copyright Executive Physical Therapy, Inc., 1996. 1-800-530-6878.
Reproduction of this page is permissible for instructional use only.

Standing Resistive Band Shoulder External Rotation
– B E G I N N E R –

PURPOSE: To strengthen shoulder muscles.

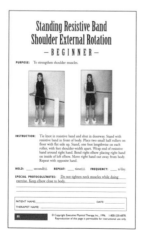

INSTRUCTION: Tie knot in resistive band and shut in doorway. Stand with resistive band in front of body. Place two small half rollers on floor with flat side up. Stand, one foot lengthwise on each roller, with feet shoulder-width apart. Wrap end of resistive band around right hand. Bend right elbow placing right hand on inside of left elbow. Move right hand out away from body. Repeat with opposite hand.

HOLD: ___ second(s). **REPEAT:** ___ time(s). **FREQUENCY:** ___ x/day.

SPECIAL PROTOCOLS/NOTES: Do not tighten neck muscles while doing exercise. Keep elbow close to body.

PATIENT NAME: _____ DATE: _____
THERAPIST NAME: _____

© Copyright Executive Physical Therapy, Inc., 1996. 1-800-530-6878.
Reproduction of this page is permissible for instructional use only.

Standing B.O.I.N.G. Shoulder Internal/External Rotation
– B E G I N N E R –

PURPOSE: To strengthen arm, forearm, hand, and shoulder muscles. To improve balance reactions.

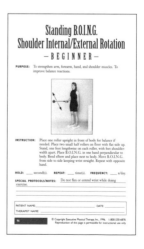

INSTRUCTION: Place one roller upright in front of body for balance if needed. Place two small half rollers on floor with flat side up. Stand, one foot lengthwise on each roller, with feet shoulder-width apart. Place B.O.I.N.G. in one hand perpendicular to body. Bend elbow and place next to body. Move B.O.I.N.G. from side to side keeping wrist straight. Repeat with opposite hand.

HOLD: ___ second(s). **REPEAT:** ___ time(s). **FREQUENCY:** ___ x/day.

SPECIAL PROTOCOLS/NOTES: Do not flex or extend wrist while doing exercise.

PATIENT NAME: _____ DATE: _____
THERAPIST NAME: _____

© Copyright Executive Physical Therapy, Inc., 1996. 1-800-530-6878.
Reproduction of this page is permissible for instructional use only.

CERVICAL STRAIN/WHIPLASH

Cervical strain or whiplash commonly occurs as a result of a motor vehicle accident. Initially, pain and swelling may be prevalent in the cervical region. Mobilize soft tissue when indicated and apply the appropriate modality to reduce swelling. At times when symptoms are acute, try strengthening the patient's cervical region indirectly, i.e., try a supine hip hike exercise to provide indirect range of motion, strengthening the scalenes and sternocleidomastoid muscles. Progress to direct range of motion and strengthening exercises.

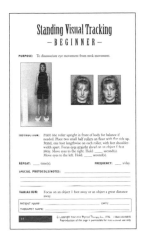

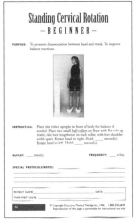

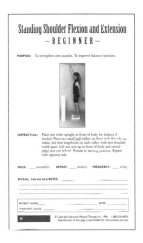

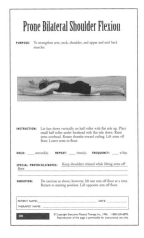

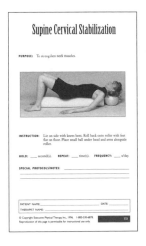

LOW BACK PAIN

More than 80% of the population experiences low back pain at some time in their life. Lumbar strain, facet dysfunction, and herniated discs can all contribute to low back pain. Evaluate the patient and determine etiology of low back pain. If inflammation is prevalent, apply the appropriate modality to low back region to reduce swelling. If indicated, instruct the patient in thoracic, lumbar, and lower extremity stretches. Progress to abdominal and lumbar strengthening exercises.

Standing Low Back Mobilization

PURPOSE: To increase range of motion in low back.

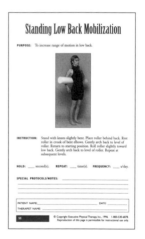

INSTRUCTION: Stand with knees slightly bent. Place roller behind back. Rest roller in crook of bent elbows. Gently arch back to level of roller. Return to starting position. Roll roller slightly toward low back. Gently arch back to level of roller. Repeat at subsequent levels.

HOLD: ___ second(s).   **REPEAT:** ___ time(s).   **FREQUENCY:** ___ x/day.

SPECIAL PROTOCOLS/NOTES: _____

PATIENT NAME: _____ DATE: _____
THERAPIST NAME: _____

© Copyright Executive Physical Therapy, Inc., 1996. 1-800-530-6878.
Reproduction of this page is permissible for instructional use only.

Cat Back Stretch I

PURPOSE: To stretch back muscles.

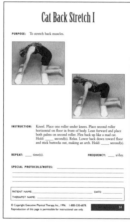

INSTRUCTION: Kneel. Place one roller under knees. Place second roller horizontal on floor in front of body. Lean forward and place both palms on second roller. Flex back up like a mad cat. Hold ___ second(s). Relax. Lower back down toward floor and stick buttocks out, making an arch. Hold ___ second(s).

REPEAT: ___ time(s).

SPECIAL PROTOCOLS/NOTES: _____

PATIENT NAME: _____ DATE: _____
THERAPIST NAME: _____

© Copyright Executive Physical Therapy, Inc., 1996. 1-800-530-6878.
Reproduction of this page is permissible for instructional use only.

Supine Hamstring Stretch

PURPOSE: To stretch back of thigh muscles.

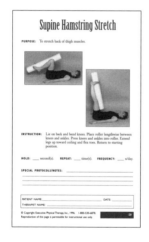

INSTRUCTION: Lie on back and bend knees. Place roller lengthwise between knees and ankles. Press knees and ankles into roller. Extend legs up toward ceiling and flex toes. Return to starting position.

HOLD: ___ second(s).   **REPEAT:** ___ time(s).   **FREQUENCY:** ___ x/day.

SPECIAL PROTOCOLS/NOTES: _____

PATIENT NAME: _____ DATE: _____
THERAPIST NAME: _____

© Copyright Executive Physical Therapy, Inc., 1996. 1-800-530-6878.
Reproduction of this page is permissible for instructional use only.

Supine Spine Stabilization 90/90

PURPOSE: To strengthen abdominal, back, and leg muscles.

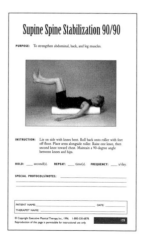

INSTRUCTION: Lie on side with knees bent. Roll back onto roller with feet off floor. Place arms alongside roller. Raise one knee, then second knee toward chest. Maintain a 90-degree angle between knees and hips.

HOLD: ___ second(s).   **REPEAT:** ___ time(s).   **FREQUENCY:** ___ x/day.

SPECIAL PROTOCOLS/NOTES: _____

PATIENT NAME: _____ DATE: _____
THERAPIST NAME: _____

© Copyright Executive Physical Therapy, Inc., 1996. 1-800-530-6878.
Reproduction of this page is permissible for instructional use only.

Supine Hip Hiker
Quadratus Lumborum Exercise

PURPOSE: To strengthen hip and low back muscles.

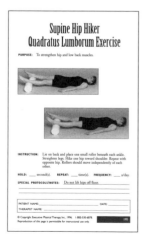

INSTRUCTION: Lie on back and place one small roller beneath each ankle. Straighten legs. Hike one hip toward shoulder. Repeat with opposite hip. Rollers should move independently of each other.

HOLD: ___ second(s).   **REPEAT:** ___ time(s).   **FREQUENCY:** ___ x/day.

SPECIAL PROTOCOLS/NOTES: _Do not lift hips off floor._

PATIENT NAME: _____ DATE: _____
THERAPIST NAME: _____

© Copyright Executive Physical Therapy, Inc., 1996. 1-800-530-6878.
Reproduction of this page is permissible for instructional use only.

PIRIFORMIS SYNDROME

The piriformis muscle is an external rotator of the hip and abductor of the hip when the knee is flexed. The sciatic nerve may run superior to, inferior to, or through the middle of the piriformis muscle. The piriformis muscle may become inflamed, tight, and painful. If inflammation exists, apply modality to the piriformis area to reduce swelling. Instruct the patient in stretching and strengthening exercises.

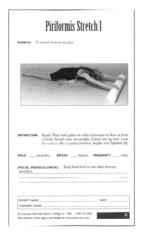

Piriformis Stretch I

PURPOSE: To stretch buttock muscles.

INSTRUCTION: Kneel. Place both palms on roller horizontal on floor in front of body. Stretch arms out straight. Extend one leg back. Lean forward as roller is pushed forward. Repeat with opposite leg.

HOLD: ___ second(s). REPEAT: ___ time(s). FREQUENCY: ___ x/day.

SPECIAL PROTOCOLS/NOTES: Keep head level so ears align between shoulders.

PATIENT NAME: ___ DATE: ___
THERAPIST NAME: ___

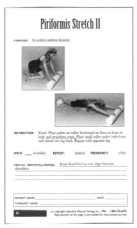

Piriformis Stretch II

PURPOSE: To stretch buttock muscles.

INSTRUCTION: Kneel. Place palms on roller horizontal on floor in front of body, and straighten arms. Place small roller under right knee and extend one leg back. Repeat with opposite leg.

HOLD: ___ second(s). REPEAT: ___ time(s). FREQUENCY: ___ x/day.

SPECIAL PROTOCOLS/NOTES: Keep head level so ears align between shoulders.

PATIENT NAME: ___ DATE: ___
THERAPIST NAME: ___

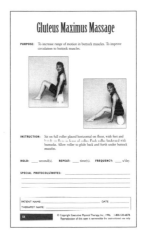

Gluteus Maximus Massage

PURPOSE: To increase range of motion in buttock muscles. To improve circulation to buttock muscles.

INSTRUCTION: Sit on full roller placed horizontal on floor, with feet and knees bent. Place hands in back of roller. Push roller backward with buttocks. Allow roller to glide back and forth under buttock muscles.

HOLD: ___ second(s). REPEAT: ___ time(s). FREQUENCY: ___ x/day.

SPECIAL PROTOCOLS/NOTES: ___

PATIENT NAME: ___ DATE: ___
THERAPIST NAME: ___

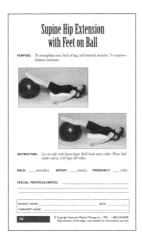

Supine Hip Extension with Feet on Ball

PURPOSE: To strengthen arm, back of leg, and buttock muscles. To improve balance reactions.

INSTRUCTION: Lie on side with knees bent. Roll back onto roller. Place ball under calves. Lift hips off roller.

HOLD: ___ second(s). REPEAT: ___ time(s). FREQUENCY: ___ x/day.

SPECIAL PROTOCOLS/NOTES: ___

PATIENT NAME: ___ DATE: ___
THERAPIST NAME: ___

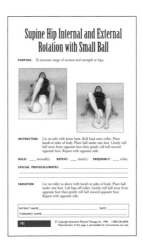

Supine Hip Internal and External Rotation with Small Ball

PURPOSE: To increase range of motion and strength in hips.

INSTRUCTION: Lie on side with knees bent. Roll back onto roller. Place hands at sides of body. Place ball under one foot. Gently roll ball away from opposite foot then gently roll ball toward opposite foot. Repeat with opposite side.

HOLD: ___ second(s). REPEAT: ___ time(s). FREQUENCY: ___ x/day.

SPECIAL PROTOCOLS/NOTES: ___

VARIATION: Lie on roller as above with hands at sides of body. Place ball under one foot. Lift hips off roller. Gently roll ball away from opposite foot then gently roll ball toward opposite foot. Repeat with opposite side.

PATIENT NAME: ___ DATE: ___
THERAPIST NAME: ___

HIP TENDONITIS

Please see case study on page 218.

PATELLOFEMORAL DYSFUNCTION

Patellofemoral Dysfunction may be caused by one or more of the following: malalignment of the patella due to weakness of the vastus medialis oblique, or tightness of the iliotibial band/gluteus medius muscle. Evaluate the patient to determine the cause of the patellofemoral dysfunction. If indicated, instruct the patient in stretching exercises for the hamstrings, quadriceps, gluteus medius, and/or iliotibial band, and strengthening exercises for the vastus medialis oblique muscle. Progress to muscle reeducation exercises so that the increased length and strength of the muscle helps the body to internalize the "normal" pattern of movement.

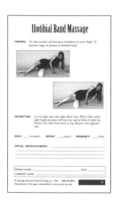

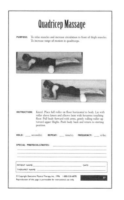

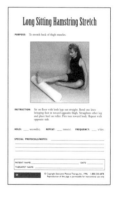

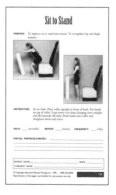

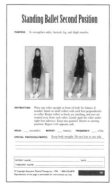

ANKLE SPRAIN

The anterior talofibular ligament is the most commonly injured ligament with ankle sprains, caused by an excessive inversion stress of the foot. Symptoms include pain, swelling, and limited ankle range of motion. Begin by administering R.I.C.E. instructions: Rest, Ice (within 24 hours of injury), Compression, and Elevation. Instruct the patient in gentle non-weight-bearing range of motion exercises and progress to weight-bearing range of motion and strengthening exercises. Please see case study on page 222.

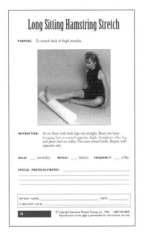

Long Sitting Hamstring Stretch

PURPOSE: To stretch back of thigh muscles.

INSTRUCTION: Sit on floor with both legs out straight. Bend one knee bringing foot in toward opposite thigh. Straighten other leg and place heel on roller. Flex toes toward body. Repeat with opposite side.

HOLD: ___ second(s). **REPEAT:** ___ time(s). **FREQUENCY:** ___ x/day.

SPECIAL PROTOCOLS/NOTES: _____

PATIENT NAME: _____ DATE: _____
THERAPIST NAME: _____

© Copyright Executive Physical Therapy, Inc., 1996. 1-800-530-6878
Reproduction of this page is permissible for instructional use only

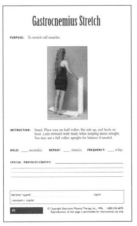

Gastrocnemius Stretch

PURPOSE: To stretch calf muscles.

INSTRUCTION: Stand. Place toes on half roller, flat side up, and heels on foot. Lean forward with body while keeping knees straight. You may use a half roller upright for balance if needed.

HOLD: ___ second(s). **REPEAT:** ___ time(s). **FREQUENCY:** ___ x/day.

SPECIAL PROTOCOLS/NOTES: _____

PATIENT NAME: _____ DATE: _____
THERAPIST NAME: _____

© Copyright Executive Physical Therapy, Inc., 1996. 1-800-530-6878
Reproduction of this page is permissible for instructional use only

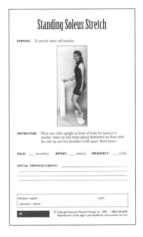

Standing Soleus Stretch

PURPOSE: To stretch inner calf muscles.

INSTRUCTION: Place one roller upright in front of body for balance if needed. Stand on half roller placed horizontal on floor with flat side up and feet shoulder-width apart. Bend knees.

HOLD: ___ second(s). **REPEAT:** ___ time(s). **FREQUENCY:** ___ x/day.

SPECIAL PROTOCOLS/NOTES: _____

PATIENT NAME: _____ DATE: _____
THERAPIST NAME: _____

© Copyright Executive Physical Therapy, Inc., 1996. 1-800-530-6878
Reproduction of this page is permissible for instructional use only

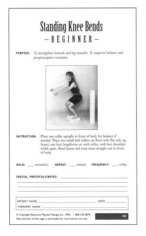

Standing Knee Bends
— BEGINNER —

PURPOSE: To strengthen buttock and leg muscles. To improve balance and proprioceptive reactions.

INSTRUCTION: Place one roller upright in front of body for balance if needed. Place two small half rollers on floor with flat side up. Stand, one foot lengthwise on each roller, with foot shoulder-width apart. Bend knees and raise arms straight out in front of body.

HOLD: ___ second(s). **REPEAT:** ___ time(s). **FREQUENCY:** ___ x/day.

SPECIAL PROTOCOLS/NOTES: _____

PATIENT NAME: _____ DATE: _____
THERAPIST NAME: _____

© Copyright Executive Physical Therapy, Inc., 1996. 1-800-530-6878
Reproduction of this page is permissible for instructional use only

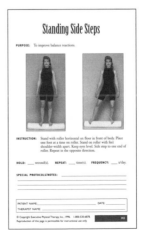

Standing Side Steps

PURPOSE: To improve balance reactions.

INSTRUCTION: Stand with roller horizontal on floor in front of body. Place one foot at a time on roller. Stand on roller with feet shoulder-width apart. Keep eyes level. Side step to one end of roller. Repeat in the opposite direction.

HOLD: ___ second(s). **REPEAT:** ___ time(s). **FREQUENCY:** ___ x/day.

SPECIAL PROTOCOLS/NOTES: _____

PATIENT NAME: _____ DATE: _____
THERAPIST NAME: _____

© Copyright Executive Physical Therapy, Inc., 1996. 1-800-530-6878
Reproduction of this page is permissible for instructional use only

CEREBROVASCULAR ACCIDENT

A cerebrovascular accident or "stroke" results when the blood supply to the brain is restricted. Multiple deficits can occur affecting motor function, sensation, mental status, perception, and language skills. Motor loss is often described as hemiplegia which occurs on the side of the body opposite the site of the lesion. Treatment for motor loss can include muscle reeducation, facilitation, positioning, and abnormal postural corrections. Treatment should focus on the areas of deficit with emphasis on normalizing function and quality of life.

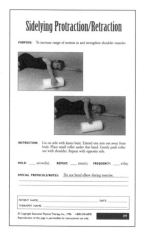

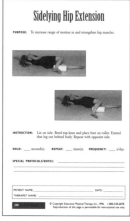

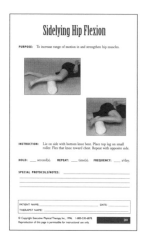

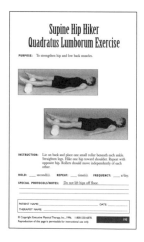

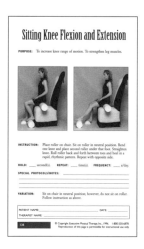

MULTIPLE SCLEROSIS

Multiple sclerosis is a demyelinating disease of the central nervous system. It mostly affects young adults and can often present with fluctuating periods of remissions and exacerbations. Clinical features of multiple sclerosis are spasticity, impaired motor function, ataxia, intention tremors, impaired sensation, visual deficits, speech problems, and bowel and bladder dysfunction. Evaluate to determine the deficit areas. Treatment focus should be to improve or at least maintain strength, motor control, coordination, gait, activities of daily living, sensory feedback, and range of motion to all joints. Treatment is most often long-term and should include an ongoing program for the patient to perform at home.

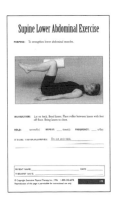

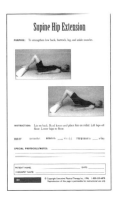

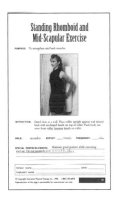

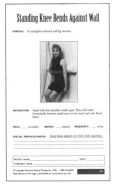

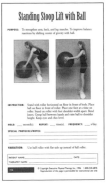

PARKINSON'S DISEASE

Parkinson's disease is a chronic progressive disease of the nervous system involving the basal ganglia. Onset usually occurs after the age of 50. Posture, balance, and gait are most commonly affected by Parkinson's disease. Treatment should focus on promoting improved posture, functional range of motion in the neck, trunk and extremities, and improving functional mobility for balance and gait.

Sitting Anterior Pelvic Tilt

PURPOSE: To increase low back range of motion. To promote neutral spine position.

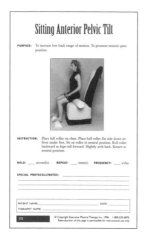

INSTRUCTION: Place full roller on chair. Place half roller flat side down on floor under feet. Sit on roller in neutral position. Roll pelvis backward as hips roll forward. Slightly arch back. Return to neutral position.

HOLD: ___ second(s). **REPEAT:** ___ time(s). **FREQUENCY:** ___ x/day.

SPECIAL PROTOCOLS/NOTES: _____

PATIENT NAME: _____ DATE: _____
THERAPIST NAME: _____

Sitting Posterior Pelvic Tilt

PURPOSE: To increase low back range of motion. To promote neutral spine position.

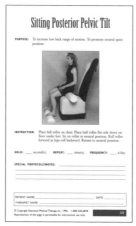

INSTRUCTION: Place full roller on chair. Place half roller flat side down on floor under feet. Sit on roller in neutral position. Roll roller forward as hips roll backward. Return to neutral position.

HOLD: ___ second(s). **REPEAT:** ___ time(s). **FREQUENCY:** ___ x/day.

SPECIAL PROTOCOLS/NOTES: _____

PATIENT NAME: _____ DATE: _____
THERAPIST NAME: _____

Sit to Stand

PURPOSE: To improve sit to stand movement. To strengthen leg and thigh muscles.

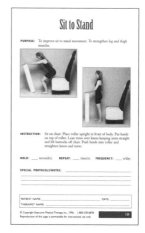

INSTRUCTION: Sit on chair. Place roller upright in front of body. Put hands on top of roller. Lean torso over knees keeping arms straight and lift buttocks off chair. Push hands into roller and straighten knees and torso.

HOLD: ___ second(s). **REPEAT:** ___ time(s). **FREQUENCY:** ___ x/day.

SPECIAL PROTOCOLS/NOTES: _____

PATIENT NAME: _____ DATE: _____
THERAPIST NAME: _____

Quadriped Upper Trunk Rotation

PURPOSE: To increase range of motion in mid and upper back, and shoulders.

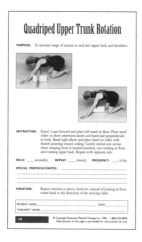

INSTRUCTION: Kneel. Lean forward and place left hand on floor. Place small roller on floor inbetween knees and hand and perpendicular to body. Bend right elbow and place hand on roller with thumb pointing toward ceiling. Gently extend arm across chest, keeping head in neutral position, eyes looking at floor, and rotating upper back. Repeat with opposite side.

HOLD: ___ second(s). **REPEAT:** ___ time(s). **FREQUENCY:** ___ x/day.

SPECIAL PROTOCOLS/NOTES: _____

VARIATION: Repeat exercise as above, however, instead of looking at floor, rotate head in the direction of the moving roller.

PATIENT NAME: _____ DATE: _____
THERAPIST NAME: _____

Quadriped Lower Trunk Rotation

PURPOSE: To increase range of motion in low back and hips.

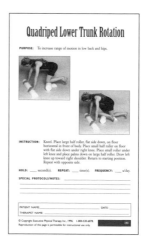

INSTRUCTION: Kneel. Place large half roller, flat side down, on floor horizontal in front of body. Place small half roller on floor with flat side down under right knee. Place small roller under left knee and place palms down on large half roller. Draw left knee up toward right shoulder. Return to starting position. Repeat with opposite side.

HOLD: ___ second(s). **REPEAT:** ___ time(s). **FREQUENCY:** ___ x/day.

SPECIAL PROTOCOLS/NOTES: _____

PATIENT NAME: _____ DATE: _____
THERAPIST NAME: _____

SWISS BALLS, RESISTIVE BANDS, and B.O.I.N.G.s

Additionally, the roller can easily be used in conjunction with other exercise equipment, such as the Swiss balls, resistive bands, and B.O.I.N.G.s, to further enhance kinesthetic and proprioceptive feedback.

The Swiss ball, also known as the Airobic ball, was originally used in the 1960s by Swiss physical therapists to help children with cerebral palsy improve their balance, reflexes, and strength. Now physical therapists and other health care professionals from around the world are teaching their clients and the general public how to break away from traditional fitness regimens and explore new strengthening, stretching, and aerobic exercises using the Swiss ball.

The following Swiss ball sizes are used throughout the book: 9 inch, 30 cm, 55 cm and 65 cm. Swiss ball exercise benefits parallel those of the foam roller exercises; however, the Swiss ball is three dimensional whereas the foam rollers are only two dimensional.

The resistive band, commonly known as Thera-band® or Dyna-Band®, is a strip of latex material designed to provide progressive resistance. Physical therapists and personal trainers routinely recommend the use of resistive bands. Thousands if not millions of people use resistive bands in their daily workouts. The versatility of the band makes it a wonderful adjunct to exercising on the foam rollers. Resistive band strips, four feet in length as used in this book, foster strength and dynamic stabilization gains.

The B.O.I.N.G. (which stands for Body Oscillation Integrates Neuromuscular Gain) was created and developed by David Greenburg, P.T., of Greenville, SC. The B.O.I.N.G. mimics rapid and repetitive muscle acceleration and deceleration performed in daily activities such as walking or throwing. In this book, one or two B.O.I.N.G.s used concurrently offer a combination of isotonic, isometric, and plyometric resistance further enhancing the dynamic stabilization effects of the foam rollers.

Notes

1. Parker, Ilana. "Beyond Conventional Exercise." *Physical Therapy Forum*, July 24, 1992, p. 4.

2. Adams, Renee. "Patient Compliance on a Roll." *P.T. Advance*, June 5, 1995, pp. 20–21.

3. Zemach-Bersin, D., Zemach-Bersin, K., & Reese, M. *Relaxercise: The Easy New Way to Health & Fitness*. New York, NY: HarperCollins Publishers, 1989.

4. Zemach-Bersin, D. per. comm.

5. Ibid.

6. Maitland, G.D. *Vertebral Manipulation: Fifth Edition*. Butterworth & Co. Ltd., 1986.

CHAPTER TWO

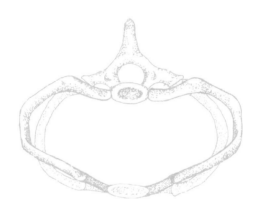

Breathing

Introduction

More than twenty thousand times per day we breathe in and out, elevating and depressing the ribs and contracting and relaxing the diaphragm and accessory muscles. Breathing in, or inhaling, exchanges air between the atmosphere and the lung aveoli, supplying body tissues with oxygen. Breathing out, or exhaling, removes carbon dioxide from the lung aveoli and transfers it to the atmosphere.

The respiratory center of the brain is located in the medulla oblongata and the pons. The medulla oblongata controls inspiration and expiration and the pons controls respiration size, pattern, and frequency. At rest, individuals without respiratory dysfunction breathe (inspiration and expiration) on average fifteen to twenty times per minute or one breath every three to four seconds.

The lung itself has no muscles to aid in the respiratory process of inhalation and exhalation, therefore, the lungs inherently expand and contract in two ways. The lungs expand with the elevation and depression of the ribs and with the inferior and superior movement of the diaphragm.

DIAPHRAGM MUSCLE

The diaphragm is the largest and most prominent muscle used in breathing. The diaphragm's dome shape separates the thoracic cavity from the abdominal cavity. The phrenic nerve which arises from the ventral rami of C3, C4, and C5[1] is the only motor supply to the diaphragm, and the sensory supply is provided by both the phrenic and intercostal nerves. The diaphragm can be controlled voluntarily by cognizance and involuntarily by the autonomic nervous system.

During inspiration, the diaphragm contracts inferiorly, lengthening the thoracic cavity vertically. Increasing the vertical dimension of the thoracic cavity creates additional space allowing the lungs to expand. During expiration, the diaphragm merely relaxes causing the elastic recoil of the lungs and the weight of the thoracic walls to compress the lungs. The diaphragm returns superiorly to its normal, relaxed position.

During exercise or heavy breathing, the inspiration process is the same as during relaxed breathing. However, the passive process of expiration is not sufficient enough to cause the essential rapid expiration necessary in heavy breathing. The additional force required during heavy breathing is exerted by the contraction of the abdominal muscles, which push superiorly against the inferior portion of the diaphragm.

RIBS

The cumulative movement of the ribs at their costotransverse joints allows for the elevation and depression of the ribs during respiration. The upper ribs, ribs one through seven, become more horizontal during inspiration creating an anteroposterior movement of the ribs and thoracic cavity (see Figure 2). The anterioposterior motion of the ribs is commonly referred to as the "pump handle" inspiratory motion (see Figure 3). The lower ribs, ribs eight

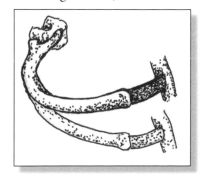

FIGURE 2

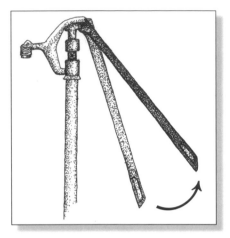

through ten, move in a lateral direction increasing the mediolateral motion and the transverse diameter of the thorax (see Figure 4). This action is commonly referred to as the "bucket handle" inspiratory motion (see Figure 5).

FIGURE 3

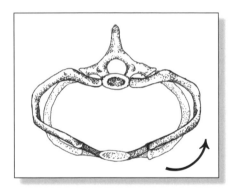

FIGURE 4

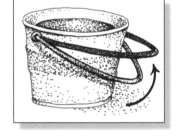

FIGURE 5

Floating ribs, ribs eleven and twelve, do not attach to the sternum and lack costotransverse joints, thereby enabling these ribs to make small movements in any direction. The quadratus lumborum muscle, however, attaches to the floating ribs, consequently limiting rib motions during inspiration.

POSTURE

Poor posture or musculoskeletal disorders can predispose individuals to respiratory dysfunction. A forward head, rounded shoulders, and trunk flexion (see Figure 6) reduce both the ability of the diaphragm to contract and the ribs to expand throughout their full range. Mellin and Harjula (1987) examined the relationship between lung function and thoracic spinal mobility and kyphosis in 272 normal individuals. They found a positive correlation between lung function (vital capacity and FEV1) and forward flexion.[2]

John Barbis states in *Rehabilitation of the Hand — Surgery and Therapy*, that poor posture predisposes patients to thoracic outlet syndrome (TOS) and "because of pain, stress, smoking, or learned habits, TOS patients can develop an abnormal breathing pattern that emphasizes upper-chest instead of diaphragmatic breathing."[3]

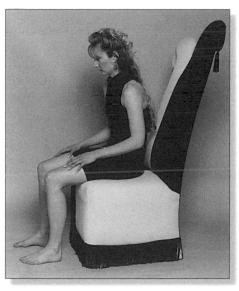

FIGURE 6

DIAPHRAGMATIC BREATHING

Breathing is rudimentary, yet paradoxically complex. We breathe every minute of our lives, yet we do not take the time to think about how we breathe. Chest breathing and shoulder breathing are the most common methods of breathing despite the fact they are incorrect.

Chest breathing involves the expansion and contraction of the chest by the pectoralis major and minor muscles. The primary muscles involved with shoulder breathing are the sternocleidomastoid, scalenus anterior, medius, and posterior muscles. Individuals with emphysema or bronchitis typically present with either chest or shoulder breathing or both. "This compromises diaphragmatic function and calls for accessory muscle use, the individual will usually exhibit an increased thoracic kyphosis protracted and internally rotated shoulders in their attempt to place the accessory muscles of respiration at a mechanical advantage."[4]

Diaphragmatic breathing involves expanding the abdomen during inhalation. The primary muscles involved with diaphragmatic breathing are the external intercostals, the transverse thoracic, and the diaphragm muscles.

Janet A. Hulme, M.A., P.T., owner of Phoenix Physical Therapy, Missoula, MT, states: "If I could teach my patients only one technique to be integrated into their daily lives, I would teach them diaphragmatic breathing." She teaches ninety percent of her patient population, which consists of fibromyalgia, headache, incontinent, and chronic pain patients, diaphragmatic breathing skills, because "diaphragmatic breathing is the foundation of what we build from, progressing to additional exercises only after instruction and successful completion of diaphragmatic breathing."

When teaching diaphragmatic breathing, the patient should

be comfortably positioned in a quiet environment. Patients should be able to breathe diaphragmatically in any position (sitting, standing, supine); however, the therapist may want to begin training in the supine position and progress to sitting and standing. Loosen clothing, belts, or any other item that may restrict the abdomen. Follow instructions on the next page for diaphragmatic breathing, and remember: the time spent inhaling should equal the time spent exhaling.

Hulme suggests diaphragmatic exercises be repeated for 30 to 60 seconds (greater than 60 seconds fatigues the muscles) every hour throughout the day to help retrain the muscles. Mark Schwartz, M.D., further recommends repeating diaphragmatic breathing exercises "during the day as part of brief relaxations" and "any time you feel physically or emotionally tense."[5]

Diaphragmatic Breathing Exercise

PURPOSE: To learn diaphragmatic breathing (abdomen expands while inhaling). To reduce muscular tension and improve breathing pattern.

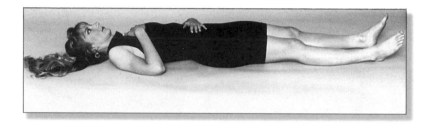

INSTRUCTION: Lie on back. Place right hand on chest and left hand on abdomen. Close eyes. Inhale through nose, extending abdomen into left hand. Hold: _____ second(s).
Exhale through mouth, as abdomen relaxes and retracts to starting position. Hold: _____ second(s).

REPEAT: _____ time(s).   **FREQUENCY:** _____ x/day.

SPECIAL PROTOCOLS/NOTES: Do not elevate chest or shoulders while
inhaling.

PATIENT NAME:_____ DATE: _____

THERAPIST NAME: _____

Notes

1. A mnemonic for remembering the ventral rami that inner-vates the diaphragm is: C3, C4, C5, Keep the Diaphragm Alive.
2. Halim, Doa. "Thoracic Spine and Rib Movements — A Dynamic Connection." *Australian Institute of Nordic Manual Therapy Newsletter*, p. I.
3. Barbis, John. *Rehabilitation of the Hand — Surgery and Therapy*. St. Louis, MO: The C.V. Mosby Company, 1995.
4. Halim, Doa. "Thoracic Spine and Rib Movements — A Dynamic Connection." *Australian Institute of Nordic Manual Therapy Newsletter*, p. I.
5. Schwartz, Mark. *Biofeedback: A Practitioners Guide*. New York: Guilford Press, 1987.

CHAPTER THREE

Computer Fitness
Guidelines

Computer fitness means more than just sitting up straight while working at your computer. Whether you are a chief executive officer or a secretarial assistant, being computer fit requires a properly positioned workstation, an ergonomic chair, nonglare lighting, and a repertoire of stretching exercises. As a result, keeping the body fit and healthy while working at a desk or computer terminal has become an ever-increasing challenge.

Desktops have become cluttered with computers, phones, fax machines, and other electronic necessities requiring workers to reach across their desks to click a mouse, bend their necks to talk on the phone, and twist their backs to type on the keyboard. Accordingly, muscular aches and pains run rampant throughout the body.

Shoulder tension, low back pain, headaches, and fatigue can all manifest from improperly arranged equipment and materials. Repetitively reaching across the desk over piles of papers to quickly grab the phone adds additional stress to overworked muscles and joints. Muscles and ligaments continue to be traumatized by slouching in a chair and typing with stiff wrists.

Jeanne Brexa, O.T.R., C.H.T., of Storage Technology Corporation, Boulder, CO, states: "Educating people on how to adjust their workstations and stretch their muscles is the best way of preventing carpal tunnel syndrome and other related injuries."

Dr. Alaina Softing, owner of PNL Vision Care, Austin, MN, reports: "100% of my clients would benefit from adjusting their workstations and taking frequent breaks from their work."

The good news is that by following the computer fitness guidelines listed below, you can reduce, if not eliminate, unwanted aches and pains.

REARRANGING YOUR WORKSTATION

Make a list prioritizing all the equipment you must use most often during the day. After finding out which items are used most frequently, place these items within 18 inches of the center of your desk. If you need to extend your arm while reaching for an object, it is too far away.

Next, adjust the computer monitor so that the top of the monitor is at eye level. If your monitor is too low, place a monitor stand or phone books under the monitor until it reaches eye level. If the monitor is too high, remove all unnecessary items from beneath the monitor. Now position the monitor so that the screen is 18–24 inches from your eyes.

Dr. Softing suggests: "Do not stare at your computer screen. Allow your eyes to become aware of objects or things happening in your peripheral vision." She also recommends: "Periodically look away from your computer screen and focus on a range of objects from far away (mountains), to near by (a picture on the wall)."

The keyboard should be positioned so that your fingers angle downward and your elbows are in line with your body. Your elbows should form angles of 90–110 degrees. If the angles of your elbows are more than 100 degrees or less than 90, you will probably need to adjust your chair.

ADJUSTING YOUR CHAIR

Sit back in your chair, with your buttocks and back firmly against the chair. If your back does not fit firmly against the backrest, you may want to lean against a McKenzie Lumbar Roll

(800) 367-7393 or a rolled-up towel.

When sitting in your chair, your knees should form a 90–100-degree angle. If your feet do not touch the floor or you have an angle greater than 100 degrees, place a footrest under your feet. You can buy a footrest, or a 3-ring binder or half of a foam roller (800) 367-7393 will work just as well. If your knees touch the top of your desk, or you have a small knee angle, then you will probably need to raise the height of your desk.

LIGHTING YOUR OFFICE

Whenever possible, light up your office with natural lighting. If direct light comes into your office, prevent it from hitting your screen by turning the shades. Angle overhead lights or lamps so the light does not glare on the screen or purchase an antiglare screen. Also, use a low wattage bulb, 60 watts or less, with a desk lamp and adjust contrast and brightness controls to allow for maximum visibility.

SPECIAL EQUIPMENT

If you find yourself talking on the phone throughout the day, you may want to purchase a telephone headset. A headset prevents shoulder and neck muscles from becoming overworked.

Do you wear bifocals or find yourself squinting at your computer monitor? You may need a new pair of eyeglasses. Computer eyeglasses are made to accommodate the 18–24-inch distance from your eyes to the screen and prevent you from tilting your head to see the screen through the bottom bifocal lens.

After adjusting your workstation, do you find that your wrists still hurt after typing for only a few minutes? If yes, try one of the new ergonomic keyboards by Ergologic (800) 665-9929 that permits the hands to type in a more natural position. Instead of typing with your palms down, you will be typing with your palms facing each other.

Need an ergonomic chair, but you're on a limited budget? Or you want to try something new? Purchase a Swiss ball to sit *and* bounce on. Physical therapists recommend that their clients get on the ball, by sitting on a ball. The round surface of the ball enables even the chronic sloucher to sit up straight.

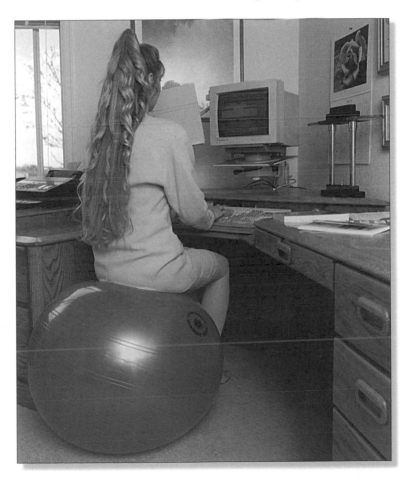

CHAPTER FOUR

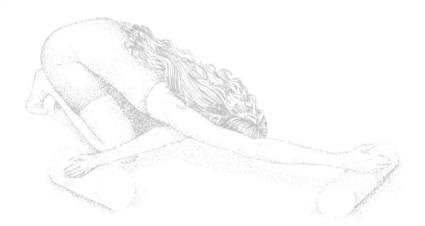

Stretching
Exercises

Stretching Exercises

Stretching Techniques

PURPOSE: To safely and effectively increase muscle length.

INSTRUCTIONS:
1. Avoid bouncing.
2. Slowly stretch into level of tolerance, not pain.
3. Do not hold your breath.
4. Repeat stretch three to five times.
5. Repeat on both sides of body.

SPECIAL PROTOCOLS/NOTES: _____

_____

_____

PATIENT NAME:_____ DATE: _____

THERAPIST NAME: _____

Wrist Flexor Stretch

PURPOSE: To stretch front side of wrist.

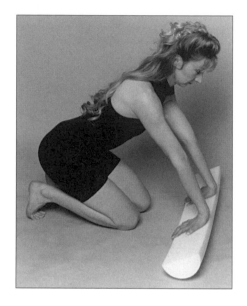

INSTRUCTION: Kneel. Place half roller, flat side up, horizontal on floor in front of body. Lean forward and place hands on half roller, palms down. Rotate hands outward so fingers point toward knees. Gently lower buttocks toward heels.

HOLD: _____ second(s).   **REPEAT:** _____ time(s).   **FREQUENCY:** _____ x/day.

SPECIAL PROTOCOLS/NOTES: _____

_____

_____

_____

PATIENT NAME:_____ DATE: _____

THERAPIST NAME: _____

Wrist Extensor Stretch

PURPOSE: To stretch back side of wrist.

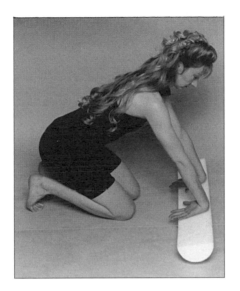

INSTRUCTION: Kneel. Place half roller, flat side, up, horizontal on floor in front of body. Lean forward and place hands on half roller, palms up. Rotate hands inward so fingers point toward knees. Gently lower buttocks toward heels.

HOLD: _____ second(s).   **REPEAT:** _____ time(s).   **FREQUENCY:** _____ x/day.

SPECIAL PROTOCOLS/NOTES: _____

_____

_____

_____

PATIENT NAME:_____ DATE: _____

THERAPIST NAME: _____

Brachioplexus Stretch

PURPOSE: To stretch shoulder and chest muscles.

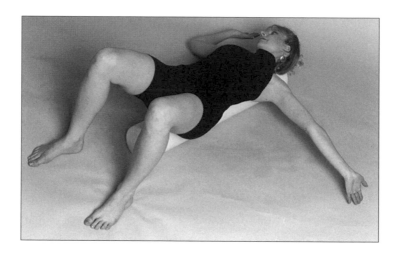

INSTRUCTION: Lie on side with knees bent. Roll back onto roller. Extend left arm and rotate arm so palm is facing up. Bend wrist back. Rotate head to right. Bend right elbow and rotate arm so palm is facing up. Repeat with opposite side.

HOLD: _____ second(s).   **REPEAT:** _____ time(s).   **FREQUENCY:** _____ x/day.

SPECIAL PROTOCOLS/NOTES: _____
_____
_____
_____

PATIENT NAME:_____ DATE: _____

THERAPIST NAME: _____

Shoulder Stretch

PURPOSE: To stretch shoulder muscles.

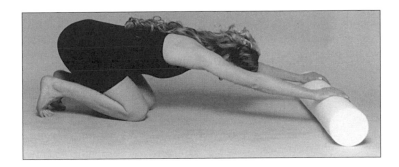

INSTRUCTION: Kneel. Sit back on heels. Roll roller away from body, keeping hands on roller and stretching arms out straight. Lower buttocks onto heels keeping ears aligned between arms.

HOLD: _____ second(s).   **REPEAT:** _____ time(s).   **FREQUENCY:** _____ x/day.

SPECIAL PROTOCOLS/NOTES: _____

_____

_____

VARIATION: Kneel. Place roller on floor horizontal in front of body. Roll roller away from body, keeping hands on roller and stretching arms out straight. Lower buttocks onto heels keeping ears aligned between arms.

PATIENT NAME:_____ DATE: _____

THERAPIST NAME: _____

Standing Shoulder Stretch

PURPOSE: To stretch arm and shoulder muscles.

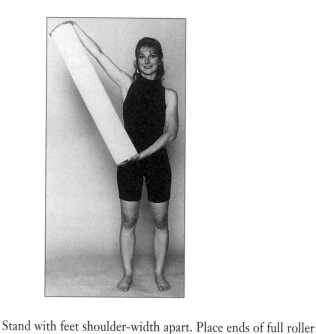

INSTRUCTION: Stand with feet shoulder-width apart. Place ends of full roller between palms of each hand. Gently move arms to the right away from body. Hold: _____ second(s). Gently move arms to the left away from body. Hold: _____ second(s).

REPEAT: _____ time(s).   **FREQUENCY:** _____ x/day.

SPECIAL PROTOCOLS/NOTES: _____

_____

_____

_____

PATIENT NAME:_____ DATE: _____

THERAPIST NAME: _____

Deltoid Stretch

PURPOSE: To stretch shoulder muscles.

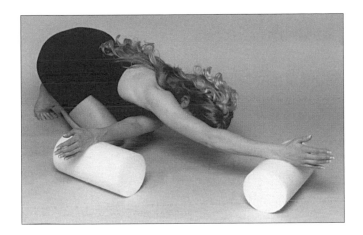

INSTRUCTION: Kneel. Straighten right arm out and place on first small roller. Reach left arm under right shoulder. Place left hand on second small roller with palm facing ceiling. Gently straighten left arm and reach toward opposite side of room. Repeat with opposite side.

HOLD: _____ second(s).   **REPEAT:** _____ time(s).   **FREQUENCY:** _____ x/day.

SPECIAL PROTOCOLS/NOTES: _____

_____

_____

_____

PATIENT NAME:_____ DATE: _____

THERAPIST NAME: _____

Thoracic and Lumbar Massage

PURPOSE: To increase range of motion in back. To improve circulation to back.

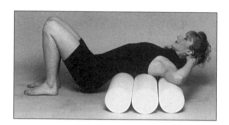

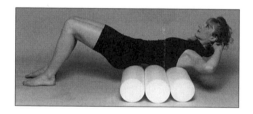

INSTRUCTION: Lie on side. Place one, two, three, or four full rollers next to upper back. Roll onto rollers. Inhale. Place unclasped hands behind head. Exhale. Gently tighten abdominal muscles as upper body rolls toward head and rollers roll toward low back. Keep body relaxed. Roll body up and down rollers.

HOLD: _____ second(s).   **REPEAT:** _____ time(s).   **FREQUENCY:** _____ x/day.

SPECIAL PROTOCOLS/NOTES: Do not arch back or pull on neck.

_____

_____

_____

PATIENT NAME:_____ DATE: _____

THERAPIST NAME: _____

Thoracic Mobilization

PURPOSE: To improve range of motion in mid back.

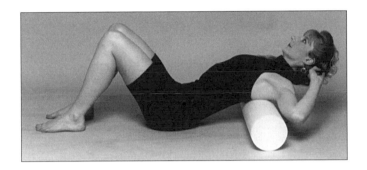

INSTRUCTION: Lie on side. Place roller horizontal to body next to upper back. Roll back onto roller with knees bent. Place feet flat on the floor. Inhale. Place unclasped hands behind head. Exhale. Gently lower head until light resistance is felt.

HOLD: _____ second(s).   **REPEAT:** _____ time(s).   **FREQUENCY:** _____ x/day.

SPECIAL PROTOCOLS/NOTES: Do not arch back or pull on neck. _____

_____

_____

_____

VARIATION: Gentle oscillations may be performed in this position with guidance from a therapist.

PATIENT NAME:_____ DATE: _____

THERAPIST NAME: _____

Standing Low Back Mobilization

PURPOSE: To increase range of motion in low back.

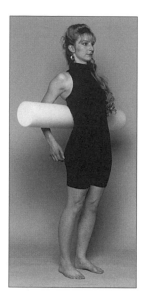

INSTRUCTION: Stand with knees slightly bent. Place roller behind back. Rest roller in crook of bent elbows. Gently arch back to level of roller. Return to starting position. Roll roller slightly toward low back. Gently arch back to level of roller. Repeat at subsequent levels.

HOLD: _____ second(s).   **REPEAT:** _____ time(s).   **FREQUENCY:** _____ x/day.

SPECIAL PROTOCOLS/NOTES: _____

_____

_____

_____

PATIENT NAME:_____ DATE: _____

THERAPIST NAME: _____

Cat Back Stretch I

PURPOSE: To stretch back muscles.

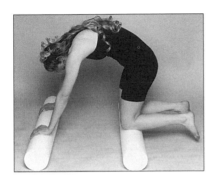

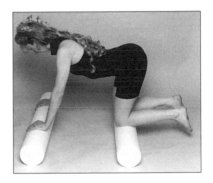

INSTRUCTION: Kneel. Place one roller under knees. Place second roller horizontal on floor in front of body. Lean forward and place both palms on second roller. Flex back up like a mad cat. Hold: _____ second(s). Relax. Lower back down toward floor and stick buttocks out, making an arch. Hold: _____ second(s).

REPEAT: _____ time(s).   **FREQUENCY:** _____ x/day.

SPECIAL PROTOCOLS/NOTES: _____

_____

_____

_____

PATIENT NAME:_____ DATE: _____

THERAPIST NAME: _____

Cat Back Stretch II

PURPOSE: To increase range of motion in back.

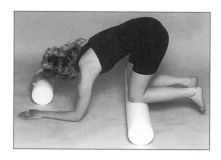

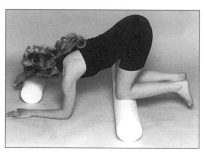

INSTRUCTION: Kneel. Place one roller under knees. Lean forward and place right palm on a small roller. Bend left elbow and place on floor. Flex back up like a mad cat. Hold: _____ second(s). Relax. Lower back down toward floor and stick buttocks out, making an arch. Hold: _____ second(s). Repeat with left palm and right elbow.

REPEAT: _____ time(s).   **FREQUENCY:** _____ x/day.

SPECIAL PROTOCOLS/NOTES: _____

_____

_____

_____

PATIENT NAME:_____ DATE: _____

THERAPIST NAME: _____

Hip Flexor Stretch

PURPOSE: To stretch front thigh and hip muscles.

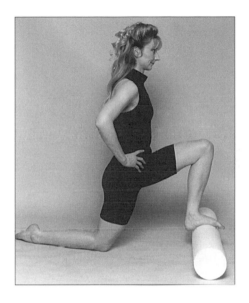

INSTRUCTION: Kneel. Place roller horizontal on floor in front of body. Place one foot on top of roller. Lean forward. Maintain a neutral spine while executing exercise. Repeat with opposite side.

HOLD: _____ second(s).   **REPEAT:** _____ time(s).   **FREQUENCY:** _____ x/day.

SPECIAL PROTOCOLS/NOTES: Do not arch or flatten back during exercise. Maintain a neutral spine.

PATIENT NAME:_____   DATE: _____

THERAPIST NAME: _____

Gluteus Maximus Massage

PURPOSE: To increase range of motion in buttock muscles. To improve circulation to buttock muscles.

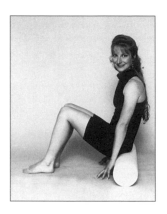

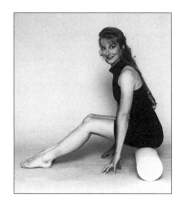

INSTRUCTION: Sit on full roller placed horizontal on floor, with feet and hands on floor in front of roller. Push roller backward with buttocks. Allow roller to glide back and forth under buttock muscles.

HOLD: ____ second(s). **REPEAT:** ____ time(s). **FREQUENCY:** ____ x/day.

SPECIAL PROTOCOLS/NOTES: _____
_____
_____
_____

PATIENT NAME:_____ DATE: _____

THERAPIST NAME: _____

Piriformis Stretch I

PURPOSE: To stretch buttock muscles.

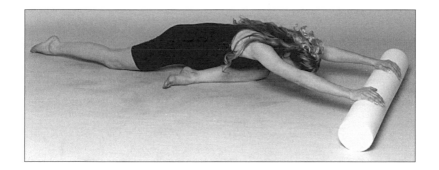

INSTRUCTION: Kneel. Place both palms on roller horizontal on floor in front of body. Stretch arms out straight. Extend one leg back. Lean forward as roller is pushed forward. Repeat with opposite leg.

HOLD: _____ second(s).   **REPEAT:** _____ time(s).   **FREQUENCY:** _____ x/day.

SPECIAL PROTOCOLS/NOTES: Keep head level so ears align between shoulders.

PATIENT NAME:_____   DATE: _____

THERAPIST NAME: _____

Piriformis Stretch II

PURPOSE: To stretch buttock muscles.

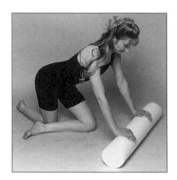

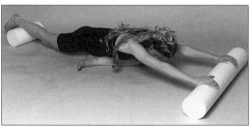

INSTRUCTION: Kneel. Place palms on roller horizontal on floor in front of body and straighten arms. Place small roller under right knee and extend one leg back. Repeat with opposite leg.

HOLD: ____ second(s).   **REPEAT:** ____ time(s).   **FREQUENCY:** ____ x/day.

SPECIAL PROTOCOLS/NOTES: Keep head level so ears align between shoulders.

_____

_____

PATIENT NAME:_____   DATE: _____

THERAPIST NAME: _____

Quadricep Massage

PURPOSE: To relax muscles and increase circulation to front of thigh muscles. To increase range of motion in quadriceps.

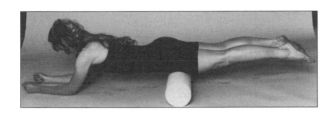

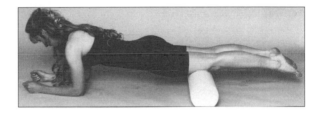

INSTRUCTION: Kneel. Place full roller on floor horizontal to body. Lie with roller above knees and elbows bent with forearms touching floor. Pull body forward with arms, gently rolling roller up toward upper thighs. Push body back and return to starting position.

HOLD: _____ second(s).   **REPEAT:** _____ time(s).   **FREQUENCY:** _____ x/day.

SPECIAL PROTOCOLS/NOTES: _____
_____
_____
_____

PATIENT NAME:_____ DATE: _____

THERAPIST NAME: _____

Long Sitting Hamstring Stretch

PURPOSE: To stretch back of thigh muscles.

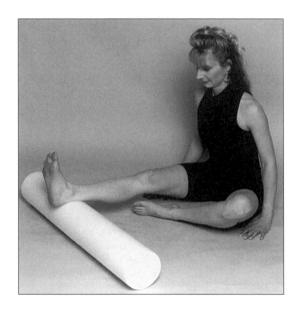

INSTRUCTION: Sit on floor with both legs out straight. Bend one knee bringing foot in toward opposite thigh. Straighten other leg and place heel on roller. Flex toes toward body. Repeat with opposite side.

HOLD: _____ second(s).   **REPEAT:** _____ time(s).   **FREQUENCY:** _____ x/day.

SPECIAL PROTOCOLS/NOTES: _____

_____

_____

_____

PATIENT NAME:_____ DATE: _____

THERAPIST NAME: _____

Supine Hamstring Stretch

PURPOSE: To stretch back of thigh muscles.

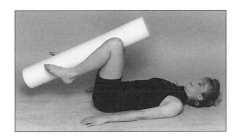

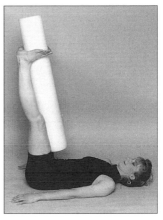

INSTRUCTION: Lie on back and bend knees. Place roller lengthwise between knees and ankles. Press knees and ankles into roller. Extend legs up toward ceiling and flex toes. Return to starting position.

HOLD: _____ second(s).　　**REPEAT:** _____ time(s).　　**FREQUENCY:** _____ x/day.

SPECIAL PROTOCOLS/NOTES: _____

_____

_____

_____

PATIENT NAME:_____ DATE: _____

THERAPIST NAME: _____

Inner Thigh Massage

PURPOSE: To increase range of motion in inner thigh. To improve circulation to inner thigh.

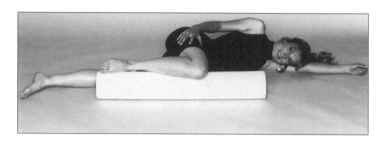

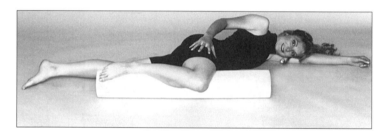

INSTRUCTION: Lie on side. Place full roller parallel to front side of body. Bend knee toward chest and place knee and foot on roller. Push roller forward with knee. Allow roller to glide down inner thigh toward groin. Return to starting position and repeat process. Repeat with opposite leg.

HOLD: _____ second(s).   **REPEAT:** _____ time(s).   **FREQUENCY:** _____ x/day.

SPECIAL PROTOCOLS/NOTES: _____

_____

_____

_____

PATIENT NAME:_____ DATE: _____

THERAPIST NAME: _____

Iliotibial Band Massage

PURPOSE: To relax muscles and increase circulation in outer thigh. To increase range of motion in iliotibial band.

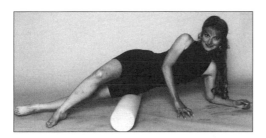

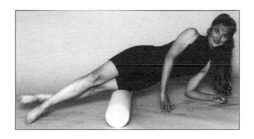

INSTRUCTION: Lie on right side with right elbow bent. Place roller under right thigh and place left leg over and in front of right leg. Gently roll roller from knee to hip. Repeat with opposite side.

HOLD: _____ second(s).   **REPEAT:** _____ time(s).   **FREQUENCY:** _____ x/day.

SPECIAL PROTOCOLS/NOTES: _____
_____
_____
_____

PATIENT NAME:_____ DATE: _____

THERAPIST NAME: _____

Gastrocnemius Stretch

PURPOSE: To stretch calf muscles.

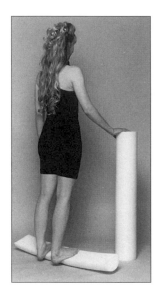

INSTRUCTION: Stand. Place toes on half roller, flat side up, and heels on floor. Lean forward with body while keeping knees straight. You may use a full roller upright for balance if needed.

HOLD: _____ second(s).   **REPEAT:** _____ time(s).   **FREQUENCY:** _____ x/day.

SPECIAL PROTOCOLS/NOTES: _____

_____

_____

_____

PATIENT NAME:_____ DATE: _____

THERAPIST NAME: _____

Sitting Soleus Stretch

PURPOSE: To stretch inner calf muscles.

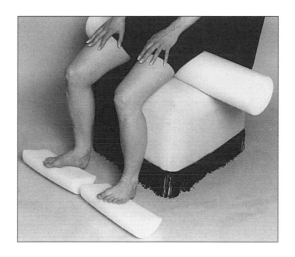

INSTRUCTION: Sit in chair. Place two small half rollers on floor with flat side up. Place feet on roller. Push heels to floor.

HOLD: _____ second(s).   **REPEAT:** _____ time(s).   **FREQUENCY:** _____ x/day.

SPECIAL PROTOCOLS/NOTES: _____
_____
_____
_____

PATIENT NAME:_____   DATE: _____
THERAPIST NAME: _____

Standing Soleus Stretch

PURPOSE: To stretch inner calf muscles.

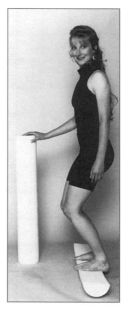

INSTRUCTION: Place one roller upright in front of body for balance if needed. Stand on half roller placed horizontal on floor with flat side up and feet shoulder-width apart. Bend knees.

HOLD: _____ second(s).   **REPEAT:** _____ time(s).   **FREQUENCY:** _____ x/day.

SPECIAL PROTOCOLS/NOTES: _____

_____

_____

_____

PATIENT NAME:_____ DATE: _____

THERAPIST NAME: _____

Anterior Foot Stretch

PURPOSE: To stretch shin muscles.

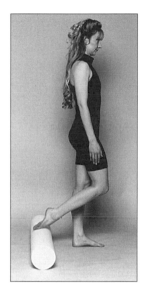

INSTRUCTION: Stand. Place full roller horizontal on floor behind body. Point toes and place one foot on top of roller so top of foot faces downward. Repeat with opposite side.

HOLD: _____ second(s).   **REPEAT:** _____ time(s).   **FREQUENCY:** _____ x/day.

SPECIAL PROTOCOLS/NOTES: _____

_____

_____

_____

PATIENT NAME:_____ DATE: _____

THERAPIST NAME: _____

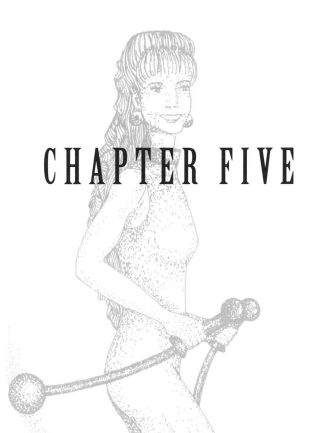

CHAPTER FIVE

Standing

Exercises

Standing Exercises

Standing Neutral Position
— BEGINNER —

PURPOSE: To strengthen muscles in an optimal position to avoid injury. To improve balance reactions.

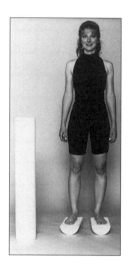

INSTRUCTION: Place one roller upright in front of body for balance if needed. Place two small half rollers on floor with flat side up. Stand, one foot lengthwise on each roller, with feet shoulder-width apart. Maintain standing with a natural curve in back. To keep balance move arms out away from body.

HOLD: _____ second(s).   **REPEAT:** _____ time(s).   **FREQUENCY:** _____ x/day.

SPECIAL PROTOCOLS/NOTES: Always begin standing exercises with a spotter to assist with balance.

_____

_____

PATIENT NAME:_____ DATE: _____

THERAPIST NAME: _____

Standing Neutral Position
— A D V A N C E D —

PURPOSE: To strengthen muscles in an optimal position to avoid injury. To improve balance reactions.

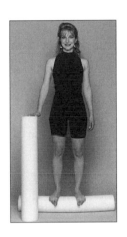 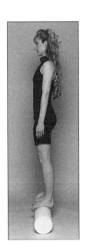

INSTRUCTION: Place one roller upright in front of body for balance if needed. Stand on second roller placed horizontal on floor with feet shoulder-width apart. Maintain standing with a natural curve in back. To keep balance, move arms out away from body.

HOLD: _____ second(s). **REPEAT:** _____ time(s). **FREQUENCY:** _____ x/day.

SPECIAL PROTOCOLS/NOTES: _____
_____
_____
_____

VARIATION: Same as above; however, stand on a half roller, flat side up.

PATIENT NAME:_____ DATE: _____
THERAPIST NAME: _____

Standing Visual Tracking
— B E G I N N E R —

PURPOSE: To disassociate eye movement from neck movement.

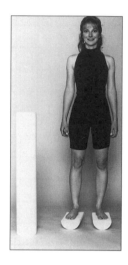
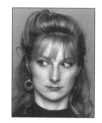
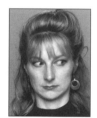

INSTRUCTION: Place one roller upright in front of body for balance if needed. Place two small half rollers on floor with flat side up. Stand, one foot lengthwise on each roller, with feet shoulder-width apart. Focus eyes straight ahead on an object 5 feet away. Move eyes to the right. Hold: _____ second(s). Move eyes to the left. Hold: _____ second(s).

REPEAT: _____ time(s).   **FREQUENCY:** _____ x/day.

SPECIAL PROTOCOLS/NOTES: _____
_____
_____
_____

VARIATION: Focus on an object 1 foot away or an object a great distance away.

PATIENT NAME:_____ DATE: _____

THERAPIST NAME: _____

Standing Visual Tracking
— A D V A N C E D —

PURPOSE: To disassociate eye movement from neck movement.

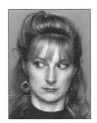 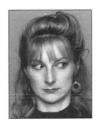 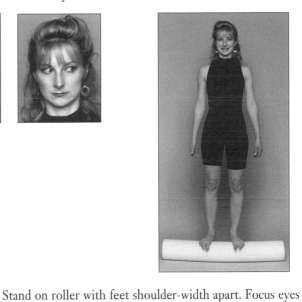

INSTRUCTION: Stand on roller with feet shoulder-width apart. Focus eyes straight ahead on an object 5 feet away.
Move eyes to the right. Hold: _____ second(s).
Move eyes to the left. Hold: _____ second(s).

REPEAT: _____ time(s).   **FREQUENCY:** _____ x/day.

SPECIAL PROTOCOLS/NOTES: _____
_____
_____
_____

VARIATION: Focus on an object 1 foot away or an object a great distance away.

PATIENT NAME:_____ DATE: _____
THERAPIST NAME: _____

Standing Cervical Rotation
– BEGINNER –

PURPOSE: To promote disassociation between head and trunk. To improve balance reactions.

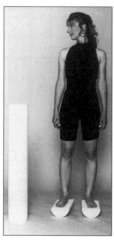

INSTRUCTION: Place one roller upright in front of body for balance if needed. Place two small half rollers on floor with flat side up. Stand, one foot lengthwise on each roller, with feet shoulder-width apart. Rotate head to right. Hold: _____ second(s). Rotate head to left. Hold: _____ second(s).

REPEAT: _____ time(s).   **FREQUENCY:** _____ x/day.

SPECIAL PROTOCOLS/NOTES: _____

_____

_____

_____

PATIENT NAME:_____ DATE: _____

THERAPIST NAME: _____

Standing Cervical Rotation
– A D V A N C E D –

PURPOSE: To promote disassociation between head and trunk. To improve balance reactions.

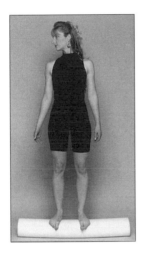 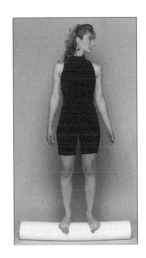

INSTRUCTION: Stand with roller horizontal on floor in front of body. Place one foot at a time on roller. Stand on roller.
Rotate head to right. Hold: _____ second(s).
Rotate head to left. Hold: _____ second(s).

REPEAT: _____ time(s).   **FREQUENCY:** _____ x/day.

SPECIAL PROTOCOLS/NOTES: _____
_____
_____
_____

PATIENT NAME:_____ DATE: _____

THERAPIST NAME: _____

Standing Shoulder Flexion
— BEGINNER —

PURPOSE: To strengthen arm muscles. To improve balance reactions.

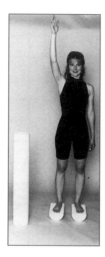

INSTRUCTION: Place one roller upright in front of body for balance if needed. Place two small half rollers on floor with flat side up. Stand, one foot lengthwise on each roller, with feet shoulder-width apart. Raise one arm overhead. Keep eyes level. Lower arm and raise opposite arm overhead.

HOLD: _____ second(s). **REPEAT:** _____ time(s). **FREQUENCY:** _____ x/day.

SPECIAL PROTOCOLS/NOTES: _____

_____

_____

_____

VARIATION: Raise one arm overhead then raise other arm overhead. Hold both overhead together for _____ second(s). Lower arms one at a time.

PATIENT NAME:_____ DATE: _____

THERAPIST NAME: _____

Standing Shoulder Flexion
– A D V A N C E D –

PURPOSE: To strengthen arm muscles. To improve balance reactions.

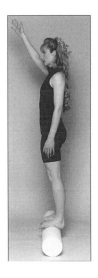

INSTRUCTION: Stand with roller horizontal on floor in front of body. Place one foot at a time on roller. Stand on roller with feet shoulder-width apart. Raise one arm overhead. Keep eyes level. Lower arm and raise opposite arm overhead.

HOLD: _____ second(s).   **REPEAT:** _____ time(s).   **FREQUENCY:** _____ x/day.

SPECIAL PROTOCOLS/NOTES: _____

_____

_____

_____

VARIATION: Raise one arm overhead then raise second arm overhead. Hold both overhead together for _____ second(s). Lower arms one at a time.

PATIENT NAME:_____ DATE: _____

THERAPIST NAME: _____

Standing Bilateral Shoulder Flexion
– BEGINNER –

PURPOSE: To strengthen arm muscles. To improve balance reactions.

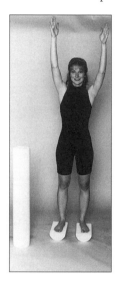

INSTRUCTION: Place one roller upright in front of body for balance if needed. Place two small half rollers on floor with flat side up. Stand, one foot lengthwise on each roller, with feet shoulder-width apart. Raise both arms overhead at same time. Keep eyes level. Lower arms to sides of body at same time.

HOLD: _____ second(s).   **REPEAT:** _____ time(s).   **FREQUENCY:** _____ x/day.

SPECIAL PROTOCOLS/NOTES: _____
_____
_____
_____

PATIENT NAME:_____ DATE: _____

THERAPIST NAME: _____

Standing Bilateral Shoulder Flexion
— A D V A N C E D —

PURPOSE: To strengthen arm muscles. To improve balance reactions.

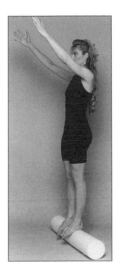

INSTRUCTION: Stand with roller horizontal on floor in front of body. Place one foot at a time on roller. Stand on roller with feet shoulder-width apart. Raise both arms overhead at same time. Keep eyes level. Lower arms to side of body at same time.

HOLD: _____ second(s).   **REPEAT:** _____ time(s).   **FREQUENCY:** _____ x/day.

SPECIAL PROTOCOLS/NOTES: _____

_____

_____

_____

PATIENT NAME:_____ DATE: _____

THERAPIST NAME: _____

Standing Shoulder Flexion and Extension
— B E G I N N E R —

PURPOSE: To strengthen arm muscles. To improve balance reactions.

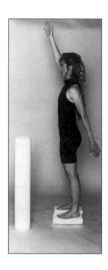

INSTRUCTION: Place one roller upright in front of body for balance if needed. Place two small half rollers on floor with flat side up. Stand, one foot lengthwise on each roller, with feet shoulder-width apart. Lift one arm up in front of body and extend other arm out behind. Return to starting position. Repeat with opposite side.

HOLD: _____ second(s).   **REPEAT:** _____ time(s).   **FREQUENCY:** _____ x/day.

SPECIAL PROTOCOLS/NOTES: _____
_____
_____
_____

PATIENT NAME:_____ DATE: _____
THERAPIST NAME: _____

Standing Shoulder Flexion and Extension
– A D V A N C E D –

PURPOSE: To strengthen arm muscles. To improve balance reactions.

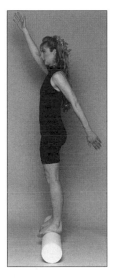

INSTRUCTION: Stand with roller horizontal on floor in front of body. Place one foot at a time on roller. Stand on roller with feet shoulder-width apart and arms down at sides of body. Lift one arm up in front of body and extend one arm out behind. Return to starting position. Repeat with opposite side.

HOLD: _____ second(s).   **REPEAT:** _____ time(s).   **FREQUENCY:** _____ x/day.

SPECIAL PROTOCOLS/NOTES: _____

_____

_____

_____

PATIENT NAME:_____ DATE: _____

THERAPIST NAME: _____

Standing Resistive Band Shoulder Flexion
– BEGINNER –

PURPOSE: To strengthen abdominal and shoulder muscles.

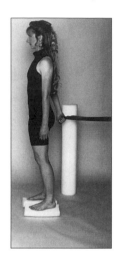 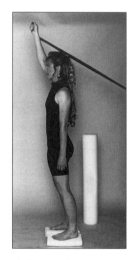

INSTRUCTION: Tie knot in resistive band and shut in doorway. Stand with resistive band behind body. Place two small half rollers on floor with flat side up. Stand, one foot lengthwise on each roller, with feet shoulder-width apart. Wrap end of resistive band around right hand. Raise right arm straight overhead, then lower to side. Repeat with opposite arm.

HOLD: _____ second(s).   **REPEAT:** _____ time(s).   **FREQUENCY:** _____ x/day.

SPECIAL PROTOCOLS/NOTES: Do not tighten neck muscles while doing exercise.

PATIENT NAME:_____ DATE: _____

THERAPIST NAME: _____

Standing Resistive Band Shoulder Flexion
– A D V A N C E D –

PURPOSE: To strengthen shoulder muscles.

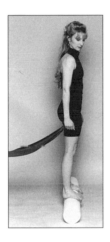 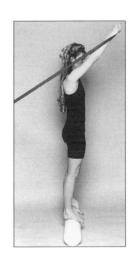

INSTRUCTION: Tie knot in resistive band and shut in doorway. Resistive band should be behind body. Stand on roller in neutral position. Wrap end of resistive band around right hand. Raise right arm straight overhead, then lower to side. Repeat with opposite arm.

HOLD: _____ second(s).   **REPEAT:** _____ time(s).   **FREQUENCY:** _____ x/day.

SPECIAL PROTOCOLS/NOTES: Do not tighten neck muscles while doing exercise.

PATIENT NAME:_____ DATE: _____

THERAPIST NAME: _____

Standing Resistive Band Shoulder Extension
— B E G I N N E R —

PURPOSE: To strengthen shoulder muscles.

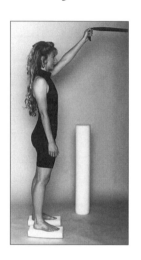 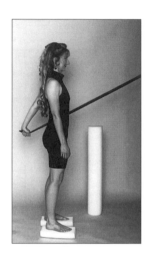

INSTRUCTION: Tie knot in resistive band and shut in doorway. Stand with resistive band behind body. Place two small half rollers on floor with flat side up. Stand, one foot lengthwise on each roller, with feet shoulder-width apart. Wrap end of resistive band around right hand. Raise right arm straight overhead, then lower to side. Repeat with opposite arm.

HOLD: _____ second(s).   **REPEAT:** _____ time(s).   **FREQUENCY:** _____ x/day.

SPECIAL PROTOCOLS/NOTES: Do not tighten neck muscles while doing exercise. _____

PATIENT NAME:_____ DATE: _____

THERAPIST NAME: _____

Standing Resistive Band Shoulder Extension
– A D V A N C E D –

PURPOSE: To strengthen shoulder muscles.

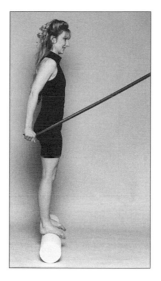

INSTRUCTION: Tie knot in resistive band and shut in doorway. Resistive band should be in front of body. Stand on roller in neutral position. Wrap end of resistive band around right hand. Raise right arm straight overhead, then lower to side. Repeat with opposite arm.

HOLD: _____ second(s).   **REPEAT:** _____ time(s).   **FREQUENCY:** _____ x/day.

SPECIAL PROTOCOLS/NOTES: Do not tighten neck muscles while doing exercise.

_____

_____

PATIENT NAME:_____   DATE: _____

THERAPIST NAME: _____

Standing Resistive Band
Shoulder Internal Rotation
– B E G I N N E R –

PURPOSE: To strengthen shoulder muscles.

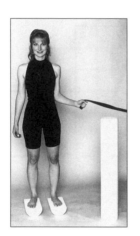 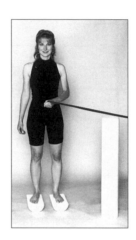

INSTRUCTION: Tie knot in resistive band and shut in doorway. Stand with resistive band in front of body. Place two small half rollers on floor with flat side up. Stand, one foot lengthwise on each roller, with feet shoulder-width apart. Wrap end of resistive band around one hand. Bend elbow and bring hand in toward abdomen. Repeat with opposite hand.

HOLD: _____ second(s).   **REPEAT:** _____ time(s).   **FREQUENCY:** _____ x/day.

SPECIAL PROTOCOLS/NOTES: Do not tighten neck muscles while doing exercise. Keep elbow close to body. _____

_____

_____

PATIENT NAME:_____ DATE: _____

THERAPIST NAME: _____

Standing Resistive Band
Shoulder Internal Rotation
– A D V A N C E D –

PURPOSE: To strengthen shoulder muscles.

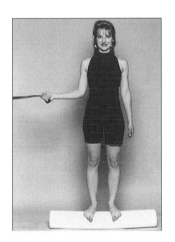 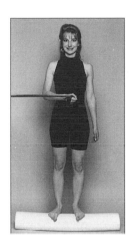

INSTRUCTION: Tie knot in resistive band and shut in doorway. Resistive band should be in front of body. Stand on roller in neutral position. Wrap end of resistive band around one hand. Bend elbow and bring hand in toward abdomen. Repeat with opposite hand.

HOLD: _____ second(s).   **REPEAT:** _____ time(s).   **FREQUENCY:** _____ x/day.

SPECIAL PROTOCOLS/NOTES: Do not tighten neck muscles while doing exercise. Keep elbow close to body.

_____

_____

PATIENT NAME:_____ DATE: _____

THERAPIST NAME: _____

Standing Resistive Band Shoulder External Rotation
– B E G I N N E R –

PURPOSE: To strengthen shoulder muscles.

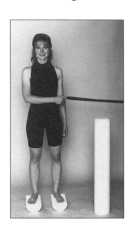 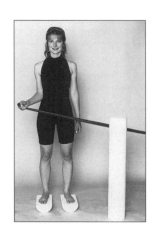

INSTRUCTION: Tie knot in resistive band and shut in doorway. Stand with resistive band in front of body. Place two small half rollers on floor with flat side up. Stand, one foot lengthwise on each roller, with feet shoulder-width apart. Wrap end of resistive band around right hand. Bend right elbow placing right hand on inside of left elbow. Move right hand out away from body. Repeat with opposite hand.

HOLD: _____ second(s).   **REPEAT:** _____ time(s).   **FREQUENCY:** _____ x/day.

SPECIAL PROTOCOLS/NOTES: Do not tighten neck muscles while doing exercise. Keep elbow close to body. _____

_____

_____

PATIENT NAME:_____ DATE: _____

THERAPIST NAME: _____

Standing Resistive Band
Shoulder External Rotation
— A D V A N C E D —

PURPOSE: To strengthen shoulder muscles.

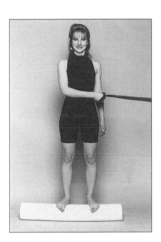
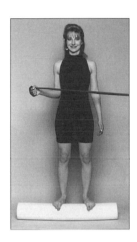

INSTRUCTION: Tie knot in resistive band and shut in doorway. Resistive band should be in front of body. Stand on roller in neutral position. Wrap end of resistive band around one hand. Bend elbow and move hand out away from body. Repeat with opposite side.

HOLD: _____ second(s). **REPEAT:** _____ time(s). **FREQUENCY:** _____ x/day.

SPECIAL PROTOCOLS/NOTES: Do not tighten muscles while doing exercise. Keep elbow close to body. _____

_____

_____

PATIENT NAME:_____ DATE: _____

THERAPIST NAME: _____

Standing Resistive Band
Shoulder PNF Diagonal One
– B E G I N N E R –

PURPOSE: To strengthen shoulder muscles.

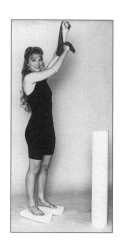 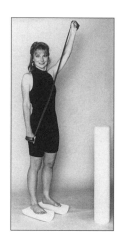

INSTRUCTION: Place two small half rollers on floor with flat side up. Stand, one foot lengthwise on each roller, with feet shoulder-width apart. Wrap ends of resistive band around each hand. Raise left arm overhead. Place right hand near left shoulder. Extend right arm down toward right thigh. Repeat with opposite side.

HOLD: ____ second(s).   **REPEAT:** ____ time(s).   **FREQUENCY:** ____ x/day.

SPECIAL PROTOCOLS/NOTES: Do not tighten neck muscles while doing exercise.

_____

_____

PATIENT NAME:_____ DATE: _____

THERAPIST NAME: _____

Standing Resistive Band
Shoulder PNF Diagonal One
– A D V A N C E D –

PURPOSE: To strengthen shoulder muscles.

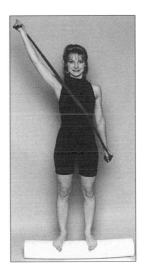

INSTRUCTION: Stand on roller in neutral position. Wrap ends of resistive band around each hand. Raise right arm overhead. Place left hand on right shoulder. Extend left arm down toward left hip. Repeat with opposite side.

HOLD: ____ second(s). **REPEAT:** ____ time(s). **FREQUENCY:** ____ x/day.

SPECIAL PROTOCOLS/NOTES: Do not tighten neck muscles while doing exercise.

PATIENT NAME:_____ DATE: _____

THERAPIST NAME: _____

Standing Resistive Band
Shoulder PNF Diagonal Two
– B E G I N N E R –

PURPOSE: To strengthen shoulder muscles.

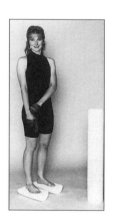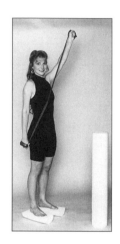

INSTRUCTION: Place two small half rollers on floor with flat side up. Stand, one foot lengthwise on each roller, with feet shoulder-width apart. Wrap ends of resistive band around each hand. Lower right hand down by right thigh. Place left hand by right thigh. Raise left hand overhead and lower. Repeat with opposite side.

HOLD: _____ second(s). **REPEAT:** _____ time(s). **FREQUENCY:** _____ x/day.

SPECIAL PROTOCOLS/NOTES: Do not tighten neck muscles while doing exercise.

_____

_____

PATIENT NAME:_____ DATE: _____

THERAPIST NAME: _____

Standing Resistive Band
Shoulder PNF Diagonal Two
– A D V A N C E D –

PURPOSE: To strengthen shoulder muscles.

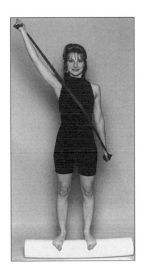

INSTRUCTION: Stand on roller in neutral position. Wrap ends of resistive band around each hand. Lower left hand down by left hip. Place right hand by left hip. Raise right hand overhead and lower. Repeat with opposite side.

HOLD: _____ second(s).   **REPEAT:** _____ time(s).   **FREQUENCY:** _____ x/day.

SPECIAL PROTOCOLS/NOTES: Do not tighten neck muscles while doing exercise.

_____

_____

PATIENT NAME:_____   DATE: _____

THERAPIST NAME: _____

Standing B.O.I.N.G.
Pronation/Supination
– BEGINNER –

PURPOSE: To strengthen arm, forearm, hand, and shoulder muscles. To improve balance reactions.

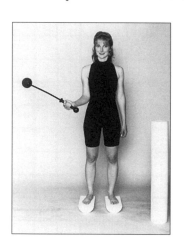 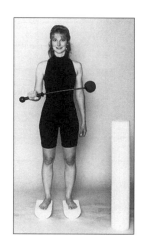

INSTRUCTION: Place one roller upright in front of body for balance if needed. Place two small half rollers on floor with flat side up. Stand, one foot lengthwise on each roller, with feet shoulder-width apart. Place B.O.I.N.G. in one hand parallel to body. Bend elbow. Move B.O.I.N.G. from side to side rotating palm up and palm down. Repeat with opposite hand.

HOLD: ____ second(s).   **REPEAT:** ____ time(s).   **FREQUENCY:** ____ x/day.

SPECIAL PROTOCOLS/NOTES: _____

_____

_____

_____

PATIENT NAME:_____ DATE: _____

THERAPIST NAME: _____

Standing B.O.I.N.G.
Pronation/Supination
— A D V A N C E D —

PURPOSE: To strengthen arm, forearm, hand, and shoulder muscles. To improve balance reactions.

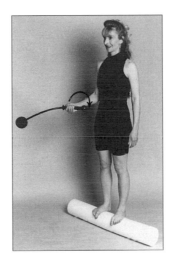

INSTRUCTION: Stand on roller. Place B.O.I.N.G. in one hand perpendicular to body. Bend elbow. Move B.O.I.N.G. from side to side rotating palm up and palm down. Repeat with opposite hand.

HOLD: _____ second(s).   **REPEAT:** _____ time(s).   **FREQUENCY:** _____ x/day.

SPECIAL PROTOCOLS/NOTES: _____

_____

_____

_____

PATIENT NAME:_____ DATE: _____

THERAPIST NAME: _____

Standing B.O.I.N.G.
Shoulder Internal/External Rotation
– BEGINNER –

PURPOSE: To strengthen arm, forearm, hand, and shoulder muscles. To improve balance reactions.

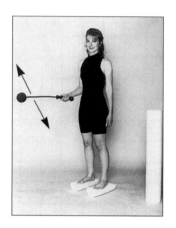

INSTRUCTION: Place one roller upright in front of body for balance if needed. Place two small half rollers on floor with flat side up. Stand, one foot lengthwise on each roller, with feet shoulder-width apart. Place B.O.I.N.G. in one hand perpendicular to body. Bend elbow and place next to body. Move B.O.I.N.G. from side to side keeping wrist straight. Repeat with opposite hand.

HOLD: _____ second(s).   **REPEAT:** _____ time(s).   **FREQUENCY:** _____ x/day.

SPECIAL PROTOCOLS/NOTES: Do not flex or extend wrist while doing exercise.

_____

_____

PATIENT NAME:_____ DATE: _____

THERAPIST NAME: _____

Standing B.O.I.N.G.
Shoulder Internal/External Rotation
– A D V A N C E D –

PURPOSE: To strengthen arm, forearm, hand, and shoulder muscles. To improve balance reactions.

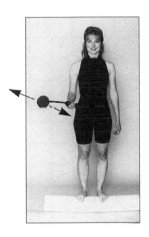

INSTRUCTION: Stand on roller placed horizontal on floor in front of body, with feet shoulder-width apart. Place B.O.I.N.G. in one hand perpendicular to body. Bend elbow and place next to body. Move B.O.I.N.G. from side to side keeping wrist straight. Repeat with opposite hand.

HOLD: _____ second(s).   **REPEAT:** _____ time(s).   **FREQUENCY:** _____ x/day.

SPECIAL PROTOCOLS/NOTES: Do not flex or extend wrist while doing _____ exercise. _____

_____

_____

PATIENT NAME:_____ DATE: _____

THERAPIST NAME: _____

Standing B.O.I.N.G. Abdominizer

PURPOSE: To strengthen abdominal and arm muscles.

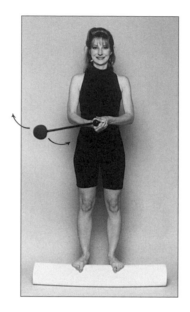

INSTRUCTION: Stand on roller. Hold B.O.I.N.G. with both hands. Extend
arms. Gently oscillate B.O.I.N.G. from side to side.

HOLD: _____ second(s).   **REPEAT:** _____ time(s).   **FREQUENCY:** _____ x/day.

SPECIAL PROTOCOLS/NOTES: _____

_____

_____

_____

PATIENT NAME:_____ DATE: _____

THERAPIST NAME: _____

Standing Rhomboid and Mid-Scapular Exercise

PURPOSE: To strengthen mid back muscles.

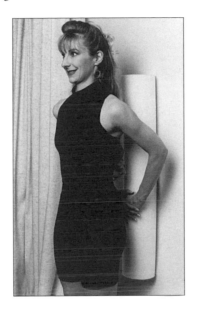

INSTRUCTION: Stand close to a wall. Place roller upright against wall behind back with unclasped hands on top of roller. Push body out away from roller, keeping hands on roller.

HOLD: _____ second(s).   **REPEAT:** _____ time(s).   **FREQUENCY:** _____ x/day.

SPECIAL PROTOCOLS/NOTES: Maintain good posture while executing exercise. Do not protrude neck or round shoulders.

_____

_____

PATIENT NAME:_____ DATE: _____

THERAPIST NAME: _____

Standing Skier with Two Rollers

PURPOSE: To improve balance reactions.

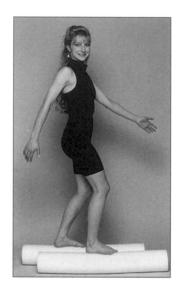

INSTRUCTION: Place two full rollers on floor parallel to each other. Stand with one foot on each roller; parallel to roller. Gently shift weight to right side of body and slide left foot and roller forward. Reach right hand forward. Repeat with opposite side, shifting weight to left side of body and sliding right foot and roller forward. Reach left hand forward.

HOLD: ____ second(s).   **REPEAT:** ____ time(s).   **FREQUENCY:** ____ x/day.

SPECIAL PROTOCOLS/NOTES: _____

_____

_____

_____

PATIENT NAME:_____ DATE: _____

THERAPIST NAME: _____

Standing B.O.I.N.G. Skier with Two Rollers

PURPOSE: To strengthen abdominal, arm, back, and leg muscles.

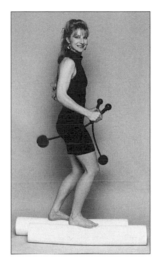

INSTRUCTION: Place two rollers on floor parallel to each other. Stand with one foot on each roller, parallel to rollers. Place one B.O.I.N.G. in each hand. Relax arms next to hips. Swing arms forward and backward as if skiing.

HOLD: _____ second(s).   **REPEAT:** _____ time(s).   **FREQUENCY:** _____ x/day.

SPECIAL PROTOCOLS/NOTES: _____

_____

_____

_____

PATIENT NAME:_____ DATE: _____

THERAPIST NAME: _____

Standing B.O.I.N.G. Skier

PURPOSE: To strengthen abdominal, arm, back, and leg muscles.

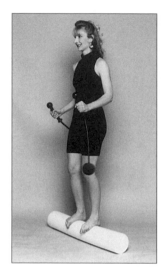

INSTRUCTION: Stand on roller horizontal on floor in front of body. Place one B.O.I.N.G. in each hand. Relax arms next to hips. Swing arms forward and backward as if skiing.

HOLD: _____ second(s).   **REPEAT:** _____ time(s).   **FREQUENCY:** _____ x/day.

SPECIAL PROTOCOLS/NOTES: _____
_____
_____
_____

VARIATION: a) Follow instructions as above; however, use one B.O.I.N.G. and swing opposite arm without a B.O.I.N.G.
b) Place two rollers on floor perpendicular to body. Stand on rollers placing right foot on one roller and left foot on the other roller. Place one B.O.I.N.G. in each hand. Relax arms next to hips. Swing arms forward and backward as if skiing.

PATIENT NAME:_____ DATE: _____

THERAPIST NAME: _____

Standing Side Steps

PURPOSE: To improve balance reactions.

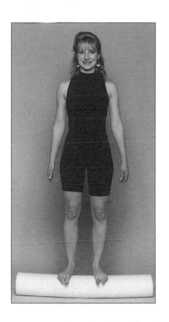 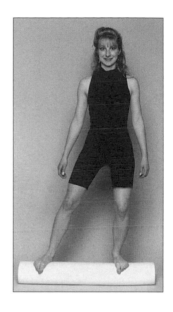

INSTRUCTION: Stand with roller horizontal on floor in front of body. Place one foot at a time on roller. Stand on roller with feet shoulder-width apart. Keep eyes level. Side step to one end of roller. Repeat in the opposite direction.

HOLD: _____ second(s).   **REPEAT:** _____ time(s).   **FREQUENCY:** _____ x/day.

SPECIAL PROTOCOLS/NOTES: _____

_____

_____

_____

PATIENT NAME:_____ DATE: _____

THERAPIST NAME: _____

Standing Side Steps with Knee Bends

PURPOSE: To strengthen buttock and leg muscles. To improve balance reactions.

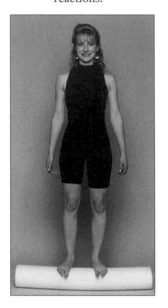 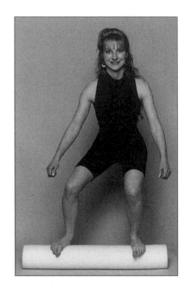

INSTRUCTION: Stand with roller horizontal on floor in front of body. Place one foot at a time on roller. Stand with feet shoulder-width apart. Side step to left. Bend knees. Stand up. Side step to right and bend knees.

HOLD: ____ second(s).   **REPEAT:** ____ time(s).   **FREQUENCY:** ____ x/day.

SPECIAL PROTOCOLS/NOTES: Keep knees aligned over feet while squatting. Do partial squat if unable to do full squat. _____
_____
_____

PATIENT NAME:_____ DATE: _____

THERAPIST NAME: _____

Standing Knee Bends
— B E G I N N E R —

PURPOSE: To strengthen buttock and leg muscles. To improve balance and proprioceptive reactions.

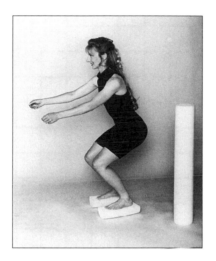

INSTRUCTION: Place one roller upright in front of body for balance if needed. Place two small half rollers on floor with flat side up. Stand, one foot lengthwise on each roller, with feet shoulder-width apart. Bend knees and raise arms straight out in front of body.

HOLD: ____ second(s).   **REPEAT:** ____ time(s).   **FREQUENCY:** ____ x/day.

SPECIAL PROTOCOLS/NOTES: _____

_____

_____

_____

PATIENT NAME:_____ DATE: _____

THERAPIST NAME: _____

Standing Knee Bends
– A D V A N C E D –

PURPOSE: To strengthen buttock and leg muscles. To improve balance and proprioceptive reactions.

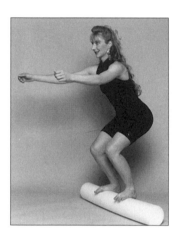 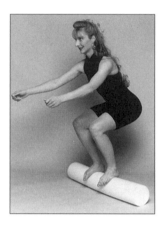

INSTRUCTION: Stand with roller horizontal on floor in front of body. Place one foot at a time on roller. Stand on roller with feet shoulder-width apart. Bend knees and raise arms out in front of body.

HOLD: ____ second(s).   **REPEAT:** ____ time(s).   **FREQUENCY:** ____ x/day.

SPECIAL PROTOCOLS/NOTES: Keep knees aligned over feet while squatting. Do partial squat and progress to full squat if unable to do full squat initially.

PATIENT NAME:_____ DATE: _____

THERAPIST NAME: _____

Standing Knee Bends Against Wall

PURPOSE: To strengthen buttock and leg muscles.

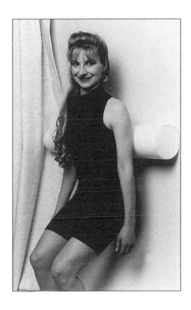

INSTRUCTION: Stand with feet shoulder-width apart. Place full roller horizontally between small curve in low back and wall. Bend knees.

HOLD: ____ second(s).   **REPEAT:** ____ time(s).   **FREQUENCY:** ____ x/day.

SPECIAL PROTOCOLS/NOTES: Keep knees aligned over feet while squatting.

_____
_____
_____

PATIENT NAME:_____   DATE: _____

THERAPIST NAME: _____

Standing Hip Hike

PURPOSE: To strengthen hip and low back muscles.

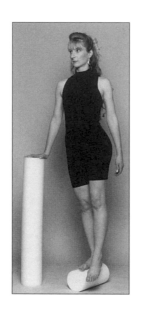 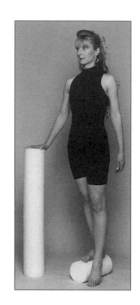

INSTRUCTION: Stand on small roller with feet parallel to roller. Lift one foot off roller and straighten leg. Slowly lower leg toward floor. Hike same hip up toward ceiling, keeping leg straight. You may use a full roller upright for balance if needed. Repeat with opposite leg.

HOLD: _____ second(s).   **REPEAT:** _____ time(s).   **FREQUENCY:** _____ x/day.

SPECIAL PROTOCOLS/NOTES: Keep body straight. Do not lean to one side. _____

_____

_____

_____

VARIATION: Use half roller instead of full roller.

PATIENT NAME:_____ DATE: _____

THERAPIST NAME: _____

Standing Ballet Second Position

PURPOSE: To strengthen ankle, buttock, leg, and thigh muscles.

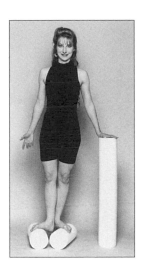 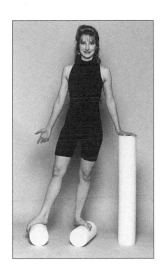

INSTRUCTION: Place one roller upright in front of body for balance if needed. Stand on small rollers with each foot perpendicular to roller. Rotate rollers so heels are touching, and toes are rotated away from each other. Gently push the roller under right foot sideways. Keep toes pointed. Return to starting position. Repeat with opposite side.

HOLD: _____ second(s). **REPEAT:** _____ time(s). **FREQUENCY:** _____ x/day.

SPECIAL PROTOCOLS/NOTES: Keep body straight. Do not lean to one side.

_____

_____

_____

PATIENT NAME:_____ DATE: _____

THERAPIST NAME: _____

Standing Ballet Fourth Position

PURPOSE: To strengthen ankle, buttock, leg, and thigh muscles.

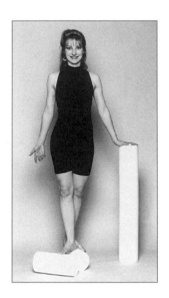 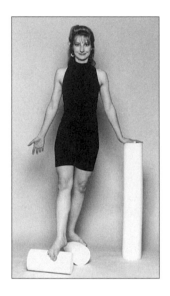

INSTRUCTION: Place one full roller upright for balance if needed. Stand on small rollers with each foot perpendicular to roller. Place right foot next to arch of left foot. Gently push the roller under right foot forward. Keep toes pointed. Return to starting position. Repeat with opposite side.

HOLD: ____ second(s).   **REPEAT:** ____ time(s).   **FREQUENCY:** ____ x/day.

SPECIAL PROTOCOLS/NOTES: Keep body straight. Do not lean to one side.

_____

_____

_____

PATIENT NAME:_____ DATE: _____

THERAPIST NAME: _____

Standing Ballet Fifth Position

PURPOSE: To strengthen ankle, buttock, leg, and thigh muscles.

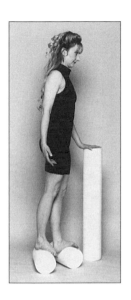 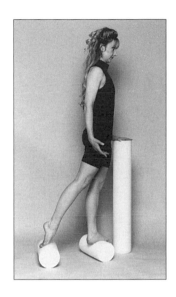

INSTRUCTION: Place one full roller upright for balance if needed. Stand on small rollers with each foot perpendicular to roller. Place right inner arch next to heel of left foot. Gently push the roller under right foot backward. Keep toes pointed. Return to starting position. Repeat with opposite side.

HOLD: _____ second(s).   **REPEAT:** _____ time(s).   **FREQUENCY:** _____ x/day.

SPECIAL PROTOCOLS/NOTES: Keep body straight. Do not lean to one side.

_____
_____
_____

PATIENT NAME:_____   DATE: _____

THERAPIST NAME: _____

Standing Stoop Lift with Ball

PURPOSE: To strengthen arm, back, and leg muscles. To improve balance reactions by shifting center of gravity with ball.

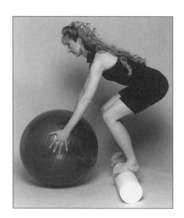 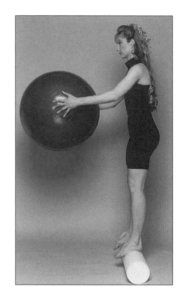

INSTRUCTION: Stand with roller horizontal on floor in front of body. Place ball on floor in front of roller. Place one foot at a time on roller. Stand on roller with feet shoulder-width apart. Bend knees. Grasp ball between hands and raise ball to shoulder height. Keep eyes and chin level.

HOLD: _____ second(s).   **REPEAT:** _____ time(s).   **FREQUENCY:** _____ x/day.

SPECIAL PROTOCOLS/NOTES: _____

_____

_____

_____

VARIATION: Use half roller with flat side up instead of full roller.

PATIENT NAME:_____ DATE: _____

THERAPIST NAME: _____

Standing Stoop to Overhead Lift with Ball

PURPOSE: To strengthen arm, back, and leg muscles. To improve balance reactions by shifting center of gravity with ball.

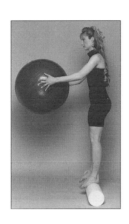 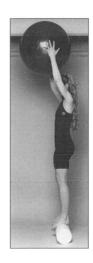

INSTRUCTION: Stand with roller horizontal on floor in front of body. Place ball on floor in front of roller. Place one foot at a time on roller. Stand on roller with feet shoulder-width apart. Begin in stoop position with ball between hands. Shift weight backward and lift ball to shoulder height. Raise ball overhead. Keep eyes and chin level.

HOLD: _____ second(s).　**REPEAT:** _____ time(s).　**FREQUENCY:** _____ x/day.

SPECIAL PROTOCOLS/NOTES:　Do not look up at ball while ball is overhead. Eyes should be looking forward at all times.

VARIATION: Use half roller with flat side up instead of full roller.

PATIENT NAME:_____ DATE: _____

THERAPIST NAME: _____

Standing Shoulder to Overhead Lift with Ball

PURPOSE: To strengthen arm, back, and leg muscles. To improve balance reactions by shifting center of gravity.

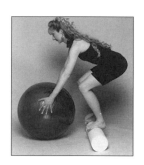 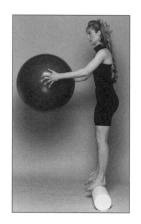 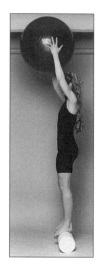

INSTRUCTION: Stand with roller horizontal on floor in front of body. Place ball on floor in front of roller. Place one foot at a time on roller. Stand on roller with feet shoulder-width apart. Bend knees. Raise ball overhead and straighten knees. Keep eyes and chin level.

HOLD: _____ second(s). **REPEAT:** _____ time(s). **FREQUENCY:** _____ x/day.

SPECIAL PROTOCOLS/NOTES: Do not look up at ball while ball is overhead. Eyes should be looking forward at all times.

VARIATION: Use half roller with flat side up instead of full roller.

PATIENT NAME:_____ DATE: _____

THERAPIST NAME: _____

Balance Beam Walk

PURPOSE: To improve balance reactions.

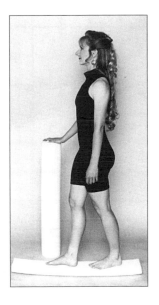

INSTRUCTION: Place one roller upright in front of body for balance if needed. Stand on full roller lengthwise with one foot in front of the other. Walk forward two steps, then backward two steps. Keep head level and eyes up.

REPEAT: _____ time(s).   **FREQUENCY:** _____ x/day.

SPECIAL PROTOCOLS/NOTES: Spotter required for this exercise.
_____
_____
_____

PATIENT NAME:_____ DATE: _____

THERAPIST NAME: _____

Standing Obstacle Course

PURPOSE: To improve balance reactions.

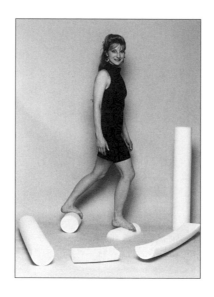

INSTRUCTION: Place one set of rollers (two 1' half rollers, two 1' full rollers, two 3' half rollers, and two 3' full rollers) on floor forming a circle. Each roller should be placed a stride's length apart from the other. Place one 3' roller upright for aiding balance. Walk on top of each roller in a clockwise direction _____ time(s) and in a counterclockwise direction _____ time(s).

FREQUENCY: _____ x/day.

SPECIAL PROTOCOLS/NOTES: Please use a spotter at all times with this exercise. _____

_____

_____

PATIENT NAME: _____ DATE: _____

THERAPIST NAME: _____

Standing Obstacle Course with Ball

PURPOSE: To improve balance reactions by shifting center of gravity with ball.

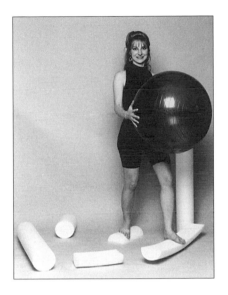

INSTRUCTION: Place one set of rollers (two 1' half rollers, two 1' full rollers, two 3' half rollers, and two 3' full rollers) on floor forming a circle. Each roller should be placed a stride's length apart from the other. Place one 3' roller upright for aiding balance. Place ball in hands. Walk on top of each roller in a clockwise direction _____ time(s) and in a counterclockwise direction _____ time(s).

FREQUENCY: _____ x/day.

SPECIAL PROTOCOLS/NOTES: Please use a spotter at all times with this exercise.

_____

PATIENT NAME:_____ DATE: _____

THERAPIST NAME: _____

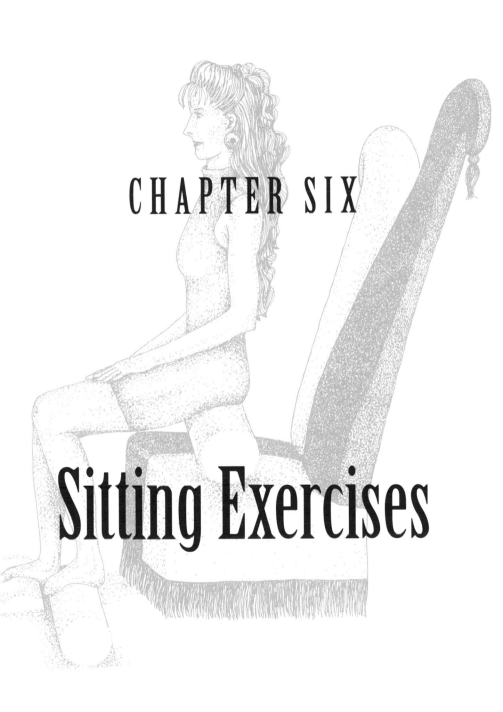

CHAPTER SIX

Sitting Exercises

Sitting Exercises

Sitting Neutral Position

PURPOSE: To strengthen muscles in an optimal position to avoid injury.

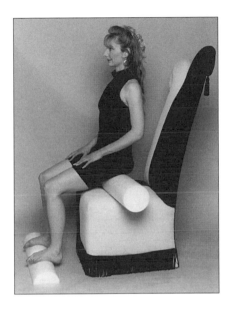

INSTRUCTION: Place full roller on chair. Place half roller flat side down on floor under feet. Sit on roller with toes pointing forward. Align knees over feet. Maintain natural curve in back.

HOLD: _____ second(s). **REPEAT:** _____ time(s). **FREQUENCY:** _____ x/day.

SPECIAL PROTOCOLS/NOTES: Do not arch or round back. _____

_____

_____

_____

PATIENT NAME:_____ DATE: _____

THERAPIST NAME: _____

Sitting Anterior Pelvic Tilt

PURPOSE: To increase low back range of motion. To promote neutral spine position.

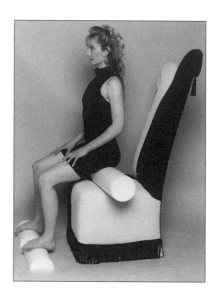

INSTRUCTION: Place full roller on chair. Place half roller flat side down on floor under feet. Sit on roller in neutral position. Roll roller backward as hips roll forward. Slightly arch back. Return to neutral position.

HOLD: _____ second(s).   **REPEAT:** _____ time(s).   **FREQUENCY:** _____ x/day.

SPECIAL PROTOCOLS/NOTES: _____

_____

_____

_____

PATIENT NAME:_____ DATE: _____

THERAPIST NAME: _____

Sitting Posterior Pelvic Tilt

PURPOSE: To increase low back range of motion. To promote neutral spine position.

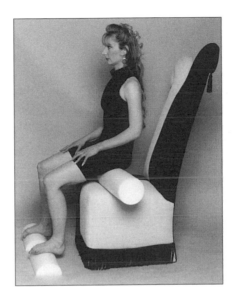

INSTRUCTION: Place full roller on chair. Place half roller flat side down on floor under feet. Sit on roller in neutral position. Roll roller forward as hips roll backward. Return to neutral position.

HOLD: _____ second(s). **REPEAT:** _____ time(s). **FREQUENCY:** _____ x/day.

SPECIAL PROTOCOLS/NOTES: _____

_____

_____

_____

PATIENT NAME:_____ DATE: _____

THERAPIST NAME: _____

Sitting Trunk Flexion

PURPOSE: To strengthen back, leg, and neck muscles. To encourage proper weight shift from sitting to standing.

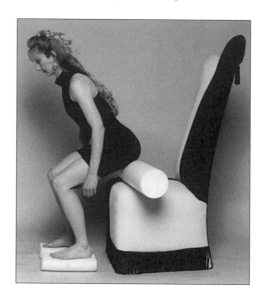

INSTRUCTION: Place full roller on chair. Sit on roller in neutral position. Place small half rollers on floor under each foot parallel to feet. Lean torso forward over knees. Return to starting position.

HOLD: ____ second(s).   **REPEAT:** ____ time(s).   **FREQUENCY:** ____ x/day.

SPECIAL PROTOCOLS/NOTES: _____

_____

_____

_____

VARIATION: Sit on chair in neutral position; however, do not sit on roller. Follow directions as above.

PATIENT NAME:_____ DATE: _____

THERAPIST NAME: _____

Sit to Stand

PURPOSE: To improve sit to stand movement. To strengthen leg and thigh muscles.

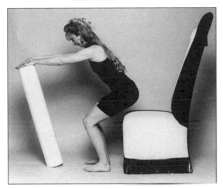

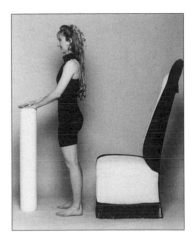

INSTRUCTION: Sit on chair. Place roller upright in front of body. Put hands on top of roller. Lean torso over knees keeping arms straight and lift buttocks off chair. Push hands into roller and straighten knees and torso.

HOLD: ____ second(s).   **REPEAT:** ____ time(s).   **FREQUENCY:** ____ x/day.

SPECIAL PROTOCOLS/NOTES: _____

_____

_____

_____

PATIENT NAME:_____ DATE: _____

THERAPIST NAME: _____

Sitting Ankle Dorsiflexion and Plantarflexion

PURPOSE: To increase range of motion in ankles.

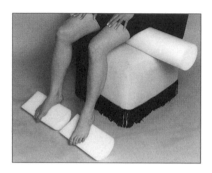

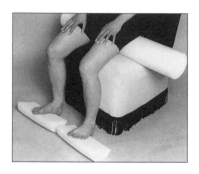

INSTRUCTION: Sit on chair. Place small half rollers on floor under each foot so rollers are parallel to feet, flat side up. Gently point and flex toes.

HOLD: _____ second(s).   **REPEAT:** _____ time(s).   **FREQUENCY:** _____ x/day.

SPECIAL PROTOCOLS/NOTES: _____

_____

_____

_____

PATIENT NAME:_____ DATE: _____

THERAPIST NAME: _____

Sitting Ankle Inversion and Eversion

PURPOSE: To increase range of motion in ankles.

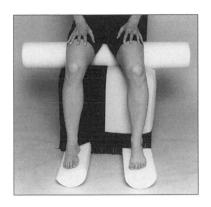

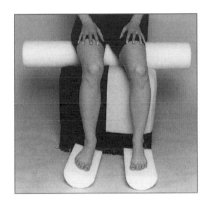

INSTRUCTION: Sit on chair. Place small half rollers on floor under both feet, flat side up. Gently move ankles from side to side.

HOLD: _____ second(s).   **REPEAT:** _____ time(s).   **FREQUENCY:** _____ x/day.

SPECIAL PROTOCOLS/NOTES: Keep knees stationary during exercise. Knees should not move from side to side with ankles.

_____

_____

PATIENT NAME:_____   DATE: _____

THERAPIST NAME: _____

Sitting Knee Flexion and Extension

PURPOSE: To increase knee range of motion. To strengthen leg muscles.

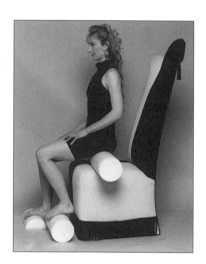 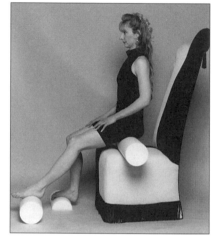

INSTRUCTION: Place roller on chair. Sit on roller in neutral position. Bend one knee and place second roller under that foot. Straighten knee. Roll roller back and forth between toes and heel in a rapid, rhythmic pattern. Repeat with opposite side.

HOLD: _____ second(s).   **REPEAT:** _____ time(s).   **FREQUENCY:** _____ x/day.

SPECIAL PROTOCOLS/NOTES: _____

_____

_____

_____

VARIATION: Sit on chair in neutral position; however, do not sit on roller. Follow instruction as above.

PATIENT NAME:_____ DATE: _____

THERAPIST NAME: _____

Long Sit Tricep Press I

PURPOSE: To strengthen muscles on back side of arm.

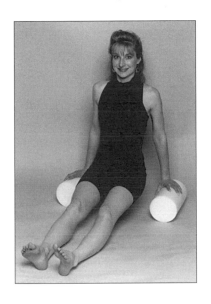
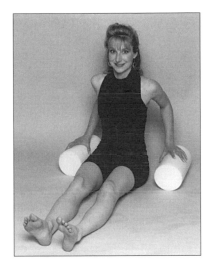

INSTRUCTION: Sit on floor with legs out straight. Place one roller on each side of hips parallel to body. Place hands on top of each roller, with thumbs on inside of roller and fingers on outside of roller. Bend elbows. Lift buttocks off floor.

HOLD: _____ second(s).   **REPEAT:** _____ time(s).   **FREQUENCY:** _____ x/day.

SPECIAL PROTOCOLS/NOTES: Do not round shoulders. _____
_____
_____
_____

PATIENT NAME:_____   DATE: _____

THERAPIST NAME: _____

Long Sit Tricep Press II

PURPOSE: To strengthen muscles on back side of arm.

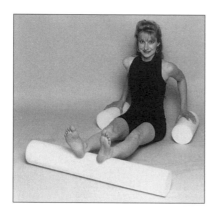
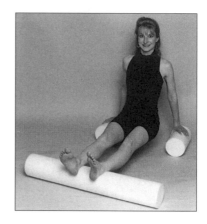

INSTRUCTION: Sit on floor with legs out straight. Place one small roller on each side of hips parallel to body and one full roller under feet. Place hands on top of each roller at sides of hips, with thumbs on inside of roller and fingers on outside of roller. Bend elbows. Lift buttocks off floor.

HOLD: _____ second(s).   **REPEAT:** _____ time(s).   **FREQUENCY:** _____ x/day.

SPECIAL PROTOCOLS/NOTES: Do not round shoulders. _____
_____
_____
_____

PATIENT NAME:_____ DATE: _____

THERAPIST NAME: _____

Long Sit Tricep Press III

PURPOSE: To strengthen muscles on back side of arm.

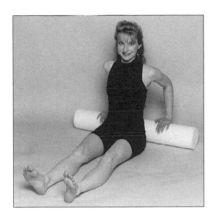

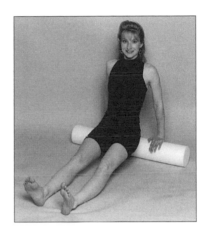

INSTRUCTION: Sit on floor with legs out straight. Place one full roller on floor behind back horizontal to body. Place hands on top of roller. Bend elbows. Lift buttocks off floor.

HOLD: _____ second(s).   **REPEAT:** _____ time(s).   **FREQUENCY:** _____ x/day.

SPECIAL PROTOCOLS/NOTES: Do not round shoulders. _____
_____
_____
_____

PATIENT NAME:_____   DATE: _____

THERAPIST NAME: _____

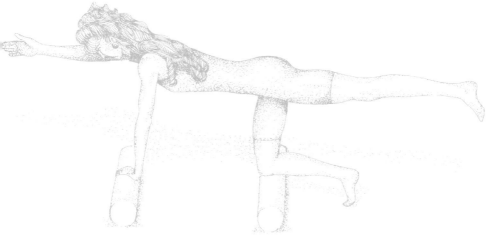

CHAPTER SEVEN

Quadriped and Kneeling Exercises

Quadriped and Kneeling Exercises

Quadriped Neutral Position

PURPOSE: To strengthen muscles in an optimal position to avoid injury.

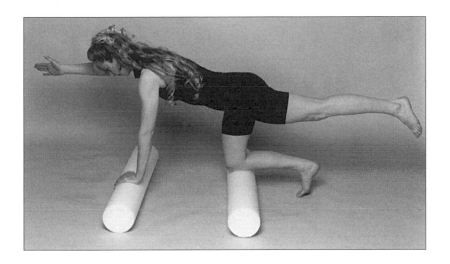

INSTRUCTION: Kneel. Place one full roller under knees. Place second full roller on floor horizontal in front of body. Lean forward and place palms on second roller. Maintain head alignment with body and natural curve in back.

HOLD: _____ second(s).   **REPEAT:** _____ time(s).   **FREQUENCY:** _____ x/day.

SPECIAL PROTOCOLS/NOTES: Do not arch or round back. _____

_____

_____

_____

PATIENT NAME:_____ DATE: _____

THERAPIST NAME: _____

Quadriped Unilateral Shoulder Flexion

PURPOSE: To strengthen arm, neck, and shoulder muscles.

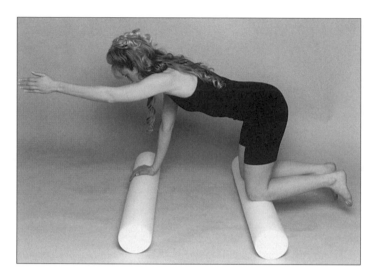

INSTRUCTION: Kneel. Place one full roller under knees. Place second full roller on floor horizontal in front of body. Lean forward and place palms on second roller. Raise one arm straight out in front. Lower arm and repeat with opposite side.

HOLD: _____ second(s). **REPEAT:** _____ time(s). **FREQUENCY:** _____ x/day.

SPECIAL PROTOCOLS/NOTES: Keep hips and back level. Do not rotate low back to do exercise.

VARIATION: Use half rollers instead of full rollers.

PATIENT NAME:_____ DATE: _____

THERAPIST NAME: _____

Quadriped Unilateral Leg Extension

PURPOSE: To strengthen back, buttock, and leg muscles.

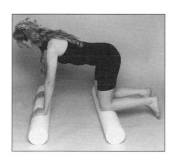

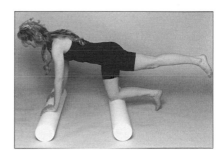

INSTRUCTION: Kneel. Place one roller under knees. Place second roller on floor horizontal in front of body. Lean forward and place palms on second roller. Extend one leg straight back. Repeat with opposite leg.

HOLD: _____ second(s). **REPEAT:** _____ time(s). **FREQUENCY:** _____ x/day.

SPECIAL PROTOCOLS/NOTES: Keep hips and back level. Do not rotate low back to do exercise.

_____

_____

_____

PATIENT NAME:_____ DATE: _____

THERAPIST NAME: _____

Quadriped Contralateral
Shoulder Flexion and Leg Extension

PURPOSE: To strengthen arm, back, neck, and leg muscles.

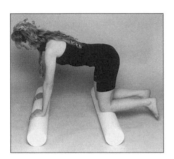

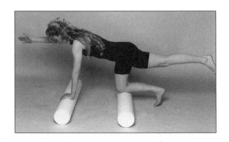

INSTRUCTION: Kneel. Place one roller under knees. Place second roller on floor horizontal in front of body. Lean forward and place palms down on roller. Raise one arm straight out in front and extend opposite leg straight back. Repeat with opposite side.

HOLD: _____ second(s).   **REPEAT:** _____ time(s).   **FREQUENCY:** _____ x/day.

SPECIAL PROTOCOLS/NOTES: Keep hips and back level. Do not rotate low back to do exercise.

_____

_____

VARIATION: Repeat exercise as above; however, raise one arm straight out in front and extend same side leg straight back.

PATIENT NAME:_____ DATE: _____

THERAPIST NAME: _____

Quadriped Hip Protraction and Retraction

PURPOSE: To strengthen hip muscles.

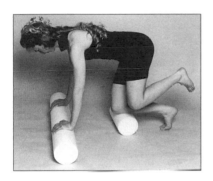
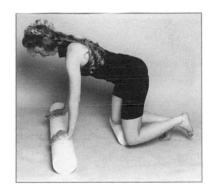

INSTRUCTION: Kneel. Place roller on floor horizontal in front of body. Lean forward and place palms down on full roller. Place small roller under right knee. Maintain neutral spine. Lift left knee off floor by contracting hip and back muscles. Keep knee aligned under hip. Return to starting position. Repeat with opposite side.

HOLD: _____ second(s).   **REPEAT:** _____ time(s).   **FREQUENCY:** _____ x/day.

SPECIAL PROTOCOLS/NOTES: Keep hips and back level. Do not arch back during exercise.

_____

_____

PATIENT NAME:_____ DATE: _____

THERAPIST NAME: _____

Quadriped Upper Trunk Rotation

PURPOSE: To increase range of motion in mid and upper back, and shoulders.

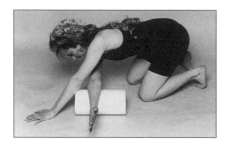

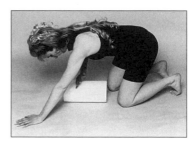

INSTRUCTION: Kneel. Lean forward and place left hand on floor. Place small roller on floor inbetween knees and hand and perpendicular to body. Bend right elbow and place hand on roller with thumb pointing toward ceiling. Gently extend arm across chest, keeping head in neutral position, eyes looking at floor, and rotating upper back. Repeat with opposite side.

HOLD: ____ second(s).   **REPEAT:** ____ time(s).   **FREQUENCY:** ____ x/day.

SPECIAL PROTOCOLS/NOTES: _____

_____

_____

_____

VARIATION: Repeat exercise as above; however, instead of looking at floor, rotate head in the direction of the moving roller.

PATIENT NAME:_____ DATE: _____

THERAPIST NAME: _____

Quadriped Lower Trunk Rotation

PURPOSE: To increase range of motion in low back and hips.

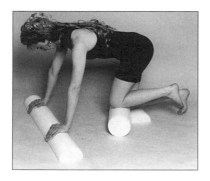

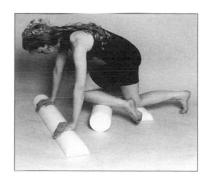

INSTRUCTION: Kneel. Place large half roller, flat side down, on floor horizontal in front of body. Place small half roller on floor with flat side down under right knee. Place small roller under left knee and place palms down on large half roller. Draw left knee up toward right shoulder. Return to starting position. Repeat with opposite side.

HOLD: _____ second(s).   **REPEAT:** _____ time(s).   **FREQUENCY:** _____ x/day.

SPECIAL PROTOCOLS/NOTES: _____

_____

_____

_____

PATIENT NAME:_____ DATE: _____

THERAPIST NAME: _____

Kneeling Neutral Position

PURPOSE: To strengthen muscles in an optimal position to avoid injury.

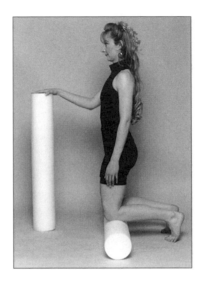

INSTRUCTION: Place one roller upright in front of body for balance if needed. Kneel on second roller placed horizontal on floor. Maintain head alignment with body and natural curve in back.

HOLD: _____ second(s).   **REPEAT:** _____ time(s).   **FREQUENCY:** _____ x/day.

SPECIAL PROTOCOLS/NOTES: Do not arch back or bend at waist. _____

_____

_____

_____

PATIENT NAME:_____ DATE: _____

THERAPIST NAME: _____

Kneeling Balance

PURPOSE: To improve balance reactions.

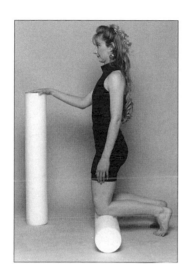 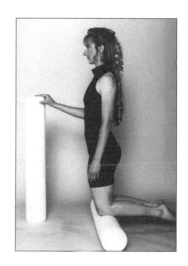

INSTRUCTION: Place one roller upright in front of body for balance if needed. Kneel on second roller placed horizontal on floor. Slowly lift toes off floor with heels pointing toward ceiling.

HOLD: _____ second(s).   **REPEAT:** _____ time(s).   **FREQUENCY:** _____ x/day.

SPECIAL PROTOCOLS/NOTES: _____

_____

_____

_____

PATIENT NAME:_____ DATE: _____

THERAPIST NAME: _____

Half Kneeling Balance
— B E G I N N E R —

PURPOSE: To strengthen leg, thigh, and trunk muscles. To improve balance reactions.

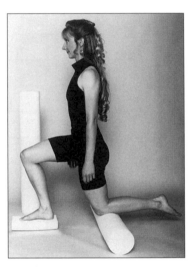

INSTRUCTION: Place one roller upright in front of body for balance if needed. Kneel on second roller placed horizontal on floor. Place small half roller, flat side up, on floor in front of body. Place right foot lengthwise on front roller. Hold: _____ second(s). Repeat with left foot. Hold: _____ second(s).

REPEAT: _____ time(s).   **FREQUENCY:** _____ x/day.

SPECIAL PROTOCOLS/NOTES: _____
_____
_____
_____

PATIENT NAME:_____ DATE: _____

THERAPIST NAME: _____

Half Kneeling Balance
— A D V A N C E D —

PURPOSE: To improve balance reactions. To strengthen leg, thigh, and trunk muscles.

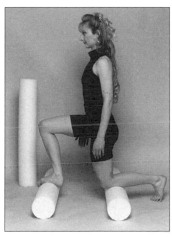

INSTRUCTION: Place one roller upright in front of body for balance if needed. Kneel on second roller placed horizontal on floor. Place third roller horizontal on floor in front of body. Place right foot on front roller. Hold: _____ second(s). Repeat with left foot. Hold: _____ second(s).

REPEAT: _____ time(s).   **FREQUENCY:** _____ x/day.

SPECIAL PROTOCOLS/NOTES: _____

_____

_____

_____

PATIENT NAME:_____ DATE: _____

THERAPIST NAME: _____

Half Kneeling Balance with Ball

PURPOSE: To improve balance reactions. To strengthen leg, thigh, and trunk muscles.

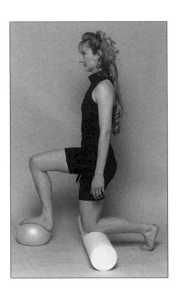

INSTRUCTION: Place one roller upright in front of body for balance if needed. Kneel on second roller placed horizontal on floor. Place small ball on floor in front of roller. Place right foot on ball. Hold: _____ second(s). Repeat with left foot. Hold: _____ second(s).

REPEAT: _____ time(s).   **FREQUENCY:** _____ x/day.

SPECIAL PROTOCOLS/NOTES: _____
_____
_____
_____

PATIENT NAME:_____ DATE: _____

THERAPIST NAME: _____

CHAPTER EIGHT

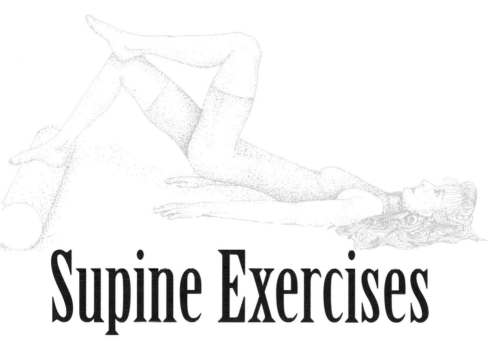

Supine Exercises

Supine Exercises

Supine Neutral Position

PURPOSE: To strengthen muscles in an optimal position to avoid injury.

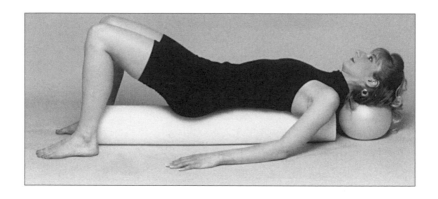

INSTRUCTION: Lie on side with knees bent. Roll back onto roller with feet flat on floor. Place small ball under head and arms alongside roller. Maintain natural curve in back

HOLD: _____ second(s).   **REPEAT:** _____ time(s).   **FREQUENCY:** _____ x/day.

SPECIAL PROTOCOLS/NOTES: Do not arch or flatten back._____

_____

_____

PATIENT NAME:_____ DATE: _____

THERAPIST NAME: _____

Supine Cervical Stabilization

PURPOSE: To strengthen neck muscles.

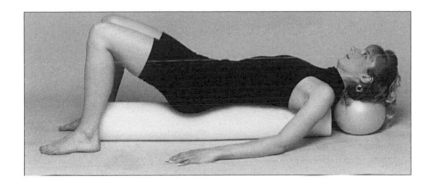

INSTRUCTION: Lie on side with knees bent. Roll back onto roller with feet flat on floor. Place small ball under head and arms alongside roller.

HOLD: ____ second(s).   **REPEAT:** ____ time(s).   **FREQUENCY:** ____ x/day.

SPECIAL PROTOCOLS/NOTES: _____
_____
_____

PATIENT NAME:_____ DATE: _____

THERAPIST NAME: _____

Supine Cervical Stabilization with Shoulder Flexion

PURPOSE: To strengthen arm and neck muscles.

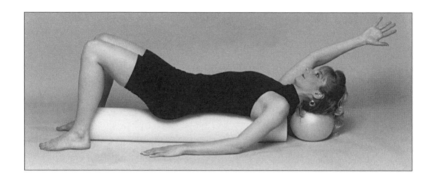

INSTRUCTION: Lie on side with knees bent. Roll back onto roller with feet flat on floor. Place small ball under head and arms alongside roller. Raise one arm overhead. Lower arm down to floor. Repeat with opposite side.

HOLD: _____ second(s). **REPEAT:** _____ time(s). **FREQUENCY:** _____ x/day.

SPECIAL PROTOCOLS/NOTES: _____
_____
_____
_____

PATIENT NAME:_____ DATE: _____

THERAPIST NAME: _____

Supine Cervical Stabilization with Knee Lift

PURPOSE: To strengthen abdominal, neck, and leg muscles.

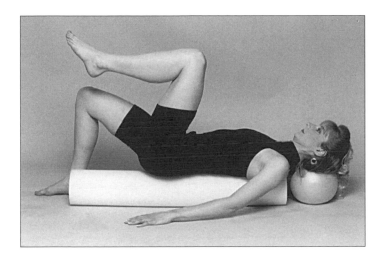

INSTRUCTION: Lie on side with knees bent. Roll back onto roller with feet flat on floor. Place small ball under head and arms alongside roller. Raise one knee, then other knee toward chest. Maintain a 90-degree angle between knees and hips.

HOLD: _____ second(s).   **REPEAT:** _____ time(s).   **FREQUENCY:** _____ x/day.

SPECIAL PROTOCOLS/NOTES: _____

_____

_____

PATIENT NAME:_____ DATE: _____

THERAPIST NAME: _____

Supine Cervical Stabilization with Shoulder and Knee Lift

PURPOSE: To strengthen abdominal, arm, leg, and neck muscles.

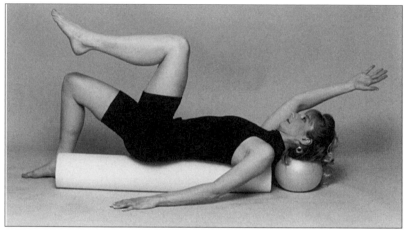

INSTRUCTION: Lie on side with knees bent. Roll back onto roller with feet flat on floor. Place small ball under head and arms alongside roller. Raise one knee, then other knee toward chest. Maintain a 90-degree angle between knees and hips.

Raise one arm overhead. Hold: _____ seconds. Lower arm to floor. Repeat with opposite arm.

REPEAT: _____ time(s).   **FREQUENCY:** _____ x/day.

SPECIAL PROTOCOLS/NOTES: _____

_____

_____

PATIENT NAME:_____ DATE: _____

THERAPIST NAME: _____

Supine Shoulder Adduction and Abduction

PURPOSE: To increase range of motion and strength in arm and shoulder muscles.

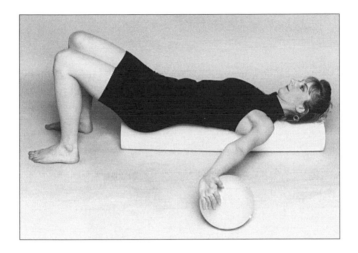

INSTRUCTION: Lie on side with knees bent. Roll back onto roller with feet flat on floor. Extend arms out to sides. Place ball under left hand. Gently roll ball up toward head and down toward hip. Repeat with opposite side.

HOLD: _____ second(s).   **REPEAT:** _____ time(s).   **FREQUENCY:** _____ x/day.

SPECIAL PROTOCOLS/NOTES: _____

_____

_____

PATIENT NAME:_____ DATE: _____

THERAPIST NAME: _____

Supine Resistive Band Shoulder Abduction

PURPOSE: To strengthen arm and chest muscles.

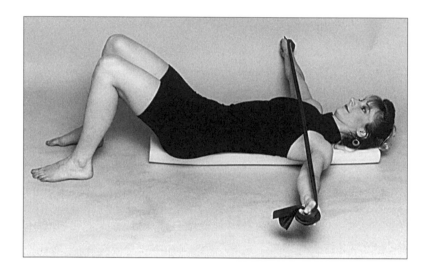

INSTRUCTION: Lie on side with knees bent. Roll back onto roller with feet flat on floor. Wrap ends of resistive band around each hand. Raise both arms toward ceiling with palms facing each other. Lower arms back down toward floor.

HOLD: _____ second(s).   **REPEAT:** _____ time(s).   **FREQUENCY:** _____ x/day.

SPECIAL PROTOCOLS/NOTES: _____
_____
_____

PATIENT NAME:_____   DATE: _____
THERAPIST NAME: _____

Supine Mid-Scapular Press

PURPOSE: To strengthen muscles between shoulder blades.

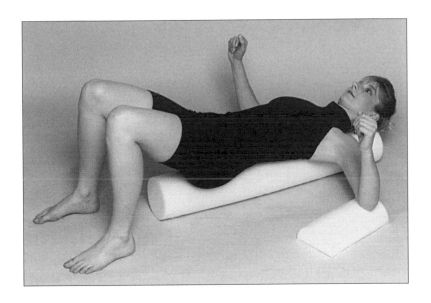

INSTRUCTION: Lie on side with knees bent. Roll back onto roller with feet flat on floor. Place elbows at approximately 70-degree angles on top of half rollers with flat sides down. Bend elbows with hands toward ceiling. Press elbows into rollers.

HOLD: _____ second(s).   **REPEAT:** _____ time(s).   **FREQUENCY:** _____ x/day.

SPECIAL PROTOCOLS/NOTES: Do not elevate shoulders toward ears during exercise.

VARIATION: As exercise becomes easier, increase elbow angles to 90 degrees.

PATIENT NAME:_____ DATE: _____

THERAPIST NAME: _____

Supine Shoulder Rolls

PURPOSE: To increase range of motion and strength in shoulder muscles.

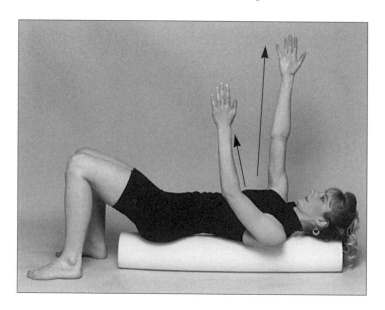

INSTRUCTION: Lie on side with knees bent. Roll back onto roller with feet flat on floor. Raise both arms with palms facing each other. Reach right hand toward ceiling as roller rolls right. Return right arm to starting position. Reach left hand toward ceiling as roller rolls left. Return left arm to starting position.

HOLD: _____ second(s).　**REPEAT:** _____ time(s).　**FREQUENCY:** _____ x/day.

SPECIAL PROTOCOLS/NOTES: _____

_____

_____

PATIENT NAME:_____ DATE: _____

THERAPIST NAME: _____

Supine Resistive Band Shoulder Rolls

PURPOSE: To increase range of motion and strength in shoulder muscles.

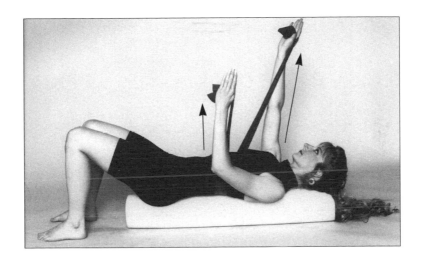

INSTRUCTION: Lie on side with knees bent. Roll back onto roller with feet flat on floor. Wrap ends of resistive band around each hand. Raise both arms toward ceiling with palms facing each other. Reach right hand toward ceiling as roller rolls right. Return right arm to starting position. Reach left hand toward ceiling as roller rolls left. Return left hand to starting position.

HOLD: _____ second(s).   **REPEAT:** _____ time(s).   **FREQUENCY:** _____ x/day.

SPECIAL PROTOCOLS/NOTES: _____
_____
_____

PATIENT NAME:_____ DATE: _____

THERAPIST NAME: _____

Supine Chest Press

PURPOSE: To strengthen arm muscles. To improve balance reactions.

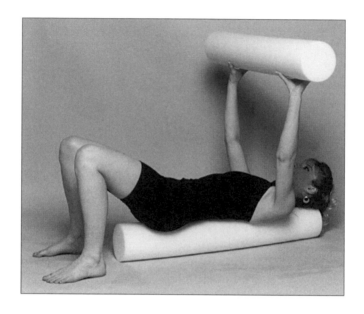

INSTRUCTION: Lie on side with knees bent. Roll back onto roller with feet flat on floor. Press second roller up toward ceiling with both hands until arms are straight up.

HOLD: _____ second(s).   **REPEAT:** _____ time(s).   **FREQUENCY:** _____ x/day.

SPECIAL PROTOCOLS/NOTES: _____

_____

_____

PATIENT NAME:_____ DATE: _____

THERAPIST NAME: _____

Supine Chest Press with Knee Lift

PURPOSE: To strengthen abdominal, arm, back, and leg muscles. To improve balance reactions.

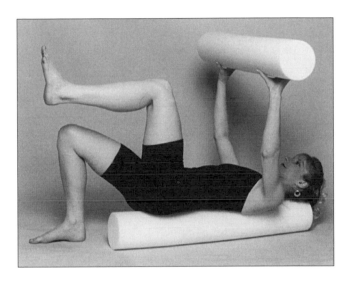

INSTRUCTION: Lie on side with knees bent. Roll back onto roller with feet flat on floor. Press second roller up toward ceiling until arms are straight while also lifting one knee. Repeat with opposite knee.

HOLD: _____ second(s).   **REPEAT:** _____ time(s).   **FREQUENCY:** _____ x/day.

SPECIAL PROTOCOLS/NOTES: _____

_____

_____

PATIENT NAME:_____ DATE: _____

THERAPIST NAME: _____

Supine Resistive Band Unilateral Shoulder Press

PURPOSE: To increase range of motion and strength in shoulder muscles.

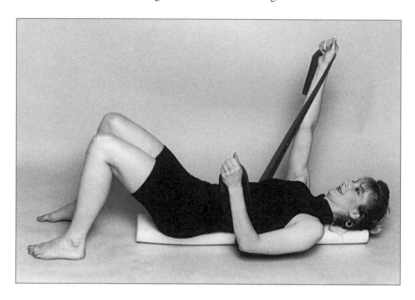

INSTRUCTION: Lie on side with knees bent. Roll back onto roller with feet flat on floor. Wrap ends of resistive band around each hand. Press right hand toward ceiling until arm is straight. Keep wrist straight during exercise. Repeat with opposite arm.

HOLD: _____ second(s).   **REPEAT:** _____ time(s).   **FREQUENCY:** _____ x/day.

SPECIAL PROTOCOLS/NOTES: _____

_____

_____

PATIENT NAME:_____ DATE: _____

THERAPIST NAME: _____

Supine Resistive Band Shoulder Press

PURPOSE: To increase range of motion and strength in shoulder muscles.

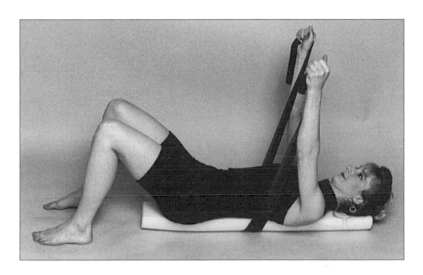

INSTRUCTION: Lie on side with knees bent. Roll back onto roller with feet flat on floor. Wrap ends of resistive band around each hand. Press both hands toward ceiling until arms are straight. Keep wrists straight during exercise.

HOLD: _____ second(s).   **REPEAT:** _____ time(s).   **FREQUENCY:** _____ x/day.

SPECIAL PROTOCOLS/NOTES: _____

_____

_____

PATIENT NAME:_____ DATE: _____

THERAPIST NAME: _____

Supine Ball Toss

PURPOSE: To strengthen arm and abdominal muscles. To promote eye-hand coordination.

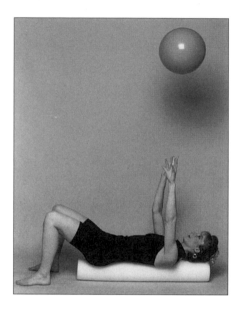

INSTRUCTION: Lie on side with knees bent. Roll back onto roller with feet flat on floor. Place ball between hands. Bend elbows. Toss ball toward ceiling. Catch ball.

REPEAT: _____ time(s).

FREQUENCY: _____ x/day.

SPECIAL PROTOCOLS/NOTES: _____

_____

_____

PATIENT NAME:_____ DATE: _____

THERAPIST NAME: _____

Supine Ball Overhead Lift

PURPOSE: To strengthen abdominal, arm, and back muscles.

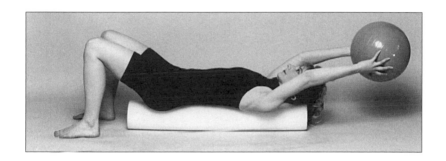

INSTRUCTION: Lie on side with knees bent. Roll back onto roller with feet flat on floor. Place ball between hands. Raise arms and ball overhead. Return to starting position.

HOLD: _____ second(s).   **REPEAT:** _____ time(s).   **FREQUENCY:** _____ x/day.

SPECIAL PROTOCOLS/NOTES: _____

_____

_____

VARIATION: Lie on side with knees bent. Roll back onto roller with feet flat on floor. Place ball between hands. Raise arms and ball overhead while lifting one knee. Return to starting position and repeat lifting opposite knee.

PATIENT NAME:_____ DATE: _____

THERAPIST NAME: _____

Supine Lower Trapezius and Mid-Scapular Exercise

PURPOSE: To strengthen muscles between shoulder blades.

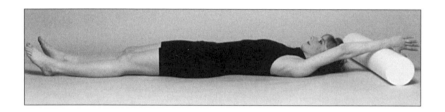

INSTRUCTION: Lie on back with legs out straight. Raise one arm overhead and place hand on top of roller. Rotate hand so thumb is pointing toward floor. Push wrist into roller. Return to starting position. Repeat with opposite side.

HOLD: _____ second(s).   **REPEAT:** _____ time(s).   **FREQUENCY:** _____ x/day.

SPECIAL PROTOCOLS/NOTES: Do not elevate shoulder toward ear during   exercise.

VARIATION: Lie with back on roller (roller is parallel to back) and bend knees. Do exercise as above.

PATIENT NAME:_____ DATE: _____

THERAPIST NAME: _____

Supine Lower Trapezius and Mid-Scapular Exercise on Roller

PURPOSE: To strengthen muscles between shoulder blades.

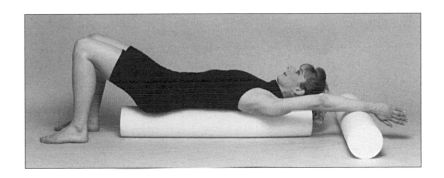

INSTRUCTION: Lie on side with knees bent. Roll back onto roller with feet flat on floor. Raise one arm overhead and place hand on top of second roller placed perpendicular to first roller. Rotate hand so thumb is pointing toward floor. Push wrist into roller. Return to starting position. Repeat with opposite arm.

HOLD: _____ second(s).   **REPEAT:** _____ time(s).   **FREQUENCY:** _____ x/day.

SPECIAL PROTOCOLS/NOTES: Do not elevate shoulder toward ear during exercise.

PATIENT NAME:_____ DATE: _____

THERAPIST NAME: _____

Supine Resistive Band PNF Diagonal One

PURPOSE: To strengthen arm, abdominal, and neck muscles.

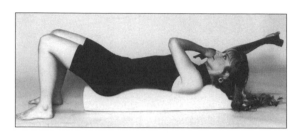

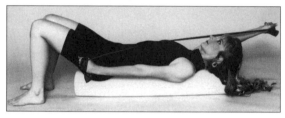

INSTRUCTION: Lie on side with knees bent. Roll back onto roller with feet flat on floor. Wrap ends of resistive band around each hand. Raise right hand toward ceiling. Place left hand on right shoulder. Extend left hand down diagonally toward left hip. Repeat with opposite arm.

HOLD: _____ second(s). **REPEAT:** _____ time(s). **FREQUENCY:** _____ x/day.

SPECIAL PROTOCOLS/NOTES: _____
_____
_____

PATIENT NAME:_____ DATE: _____

THERAPIST NAME: _____

Supine Resistive Band
PNF Diagonal Two

PURPOSE: To strengthen arm, abdominal, and neck muscles.

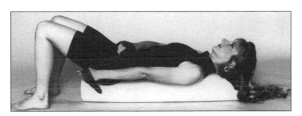

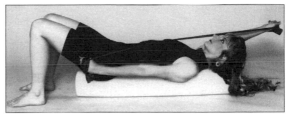

INSTRUCTION: Lie on side with knees bent. Roll back onto roller with feet flat on floor. Wrap ends of resistive band around each hand. Extend left arm toward left hip. Place right hand on left hip. Extend right arm diagonally overhead. Repeat with opposite arm.

HOLD: _____ second(s).   **REPEAT:** _____ time(s).   **FREQUENCY:** _____ x/day.

SPECIAL PROTOCOLS/NOTES: _____

_____

_____

PATIENT NAME:_____ DATE: _____

THERAPIST NAME: _____

Supine B.O.I.N.G.
Lower Trapezius Exercise

PURPOSE: To strengthen mid back muscles.

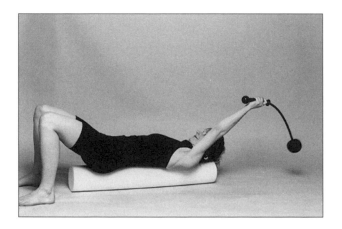

INSTRUCTION: Lie on side with knees bent. Roll back onto roller with feet flat on floor. Place B.O.I.N.G. in one hand and raise hand overhead. Gently oscillate the B.O.I.N.G. up and down, keeping the arm straight. Repeat with opposite arm.

HOLD: ____ second(s).   **REPEAT:** ____ time(s).   **FREQUENCY:** ____ x/day.

SPECIAL PROTOCOLS/NOTES: Do not tighten neck muscles while doing exercise.

VARIATIONS: a) Lie on roller. Place B.O.I.N.G. in one hand. Extend arm alongside body. Gently oscillate B.O.I.N.G. Repeat with opposite side.
b) Lie on roller. Place one B.O.I.N.G. in each hand. Extend one arm alongside body and raise opposite hand overhead. Gently oscillate both B.O.I.N.G.s at the same time. Repeat with opposite side.

PATIENT NAME:_____ DATE: _____

THERAPIST NAME: _____

Supine Resistive Band Abdominizer

PURPOSE: To strengthen abdominal, arm, and neck muscles.

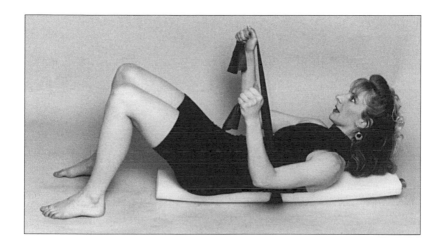

INSTRUCTION: Place resistive band under roller at mid back level. Lie on side with knees bent. Roll back onto roller with feet flat on floor. Wrap ends of resistive band around each hand. Bend elbows and place on floor. Raise head off roller while raising elbows off floor. Keep eyes on ceiling. Return to starting position.

HOLD: _____ second(s).   **REPEAT:** _____ time(s).   **FREQUENCY:** _____ x/day.

SPECIAL PROTOCOLS/NOTES: _____

_____

_____

PATIENT NAME:_____ DATE: _____

THERAPIST NAME: _____

Supine B.O.I.N.G. Abdominizer

PURPOSE: To strengthen abdominal, arm, and back muscles.

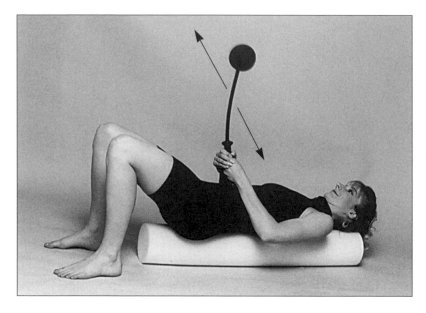

INSTRUCTION: Lie on side with knees bent. Roll back onto roller with feet flat on floor. Clasp B.O.I.N.G. in both hands and bend elbows. Gently oscillate B.O.I.N.G. from side to side.

HOLD: _____ second(s).   **REPEAT:** _____ time(s).   **FREQUENCY:** _____ x/day.

SPECIAL PROTOCOLS/NOTES: _____

_____

_____

PATIENT NAME:_____ DATE: _____

THERAPIST NAME: _____

Supine Knee Rolls on Ball

PURPOSE: To increase range of motion in low back. To strengthen abdominal oblique muscles.

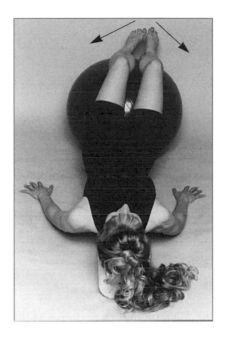

INSTRUCTION: Lie on side with knees bent. Roll back onto roller. Place ball under knees. Roll ball from side to side with knees.

HOLD: _____ second(s).   **REPEAT:** _____ time(s).   **FREQUENCY:** _____ x/day.

SPECIAL PROTOCOLS/NOTES: _____

_____

_____

PATIENT NAME:_____   DATE: _____

THERAPIST NAME: _____

Supine Leg Rolls on Ball

PURPOSE: To strengthen hip, leg, and oblique abdominal muscles.

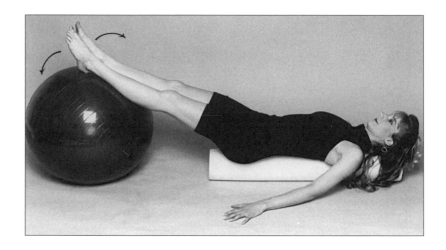

INSTRUCTION: Lie on side with knees bent. Roll back onto roller and straighten legs out. Place ball under heels. Roll ball from side to side with feet. Keep legs straight.

HOLD: ____ second(s).   **REPEAT:** ____ time(s).   **FREQUENCY:** ____ x/day.

SPECIAL PROTOCOLS/NOTES: _____

_____

_____

PATIENT NAME:_____ DATE: _____

THERAPIST NAME: _____

Supine Lower Abdominal Exercise

PURPOSE: To strengthen lower abdominal muscles.

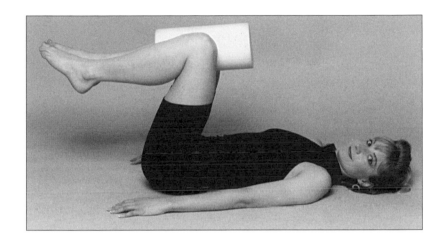

INSTRUCTION: Lie on back. Bend knees. Place roller between knees with feet off floor. Bring knees to chest.

HOLD: _____ second(s).   **REPEAT:** _____ time(s).   **FREQUENCY:** _____ x/day.

SPECIAL PROTOCOLS/NOTES: Do not arch back. _____

_____

_____

PATIENT NAME:_____   DATE: _____

THERAPIST NAME: _____

Supine Lower Abdominal Oblique Exercise

PURPOSE: To strengthen oblique abdominal muscles.

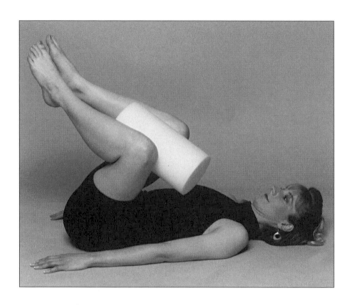

INSTRUCTION: Lie on back. Bend knees. Place roller between knees with feet off floor. Bring knees toward left shoulder. Repeat in opposite direction.

HOLD: _____ second(s).   **REPEAT:** _____ time(s).   **FREQUENCY:** _____ x/day.

SPECIAL PROTOCOLS/NOTES: Do not arch back. _____

_____

_____

PATIENT NAME:_____ DATE: _____

THERAPIST NAME: _____

Supine Unilateral Arm Raise

PURPOSE: To strengthen abdominal, arm, and back muscles.

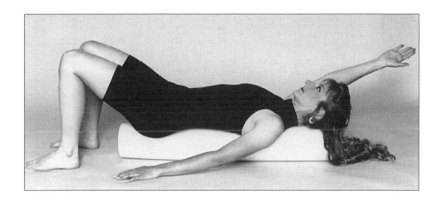

INSTRUCTION: Lie on side with knees bent. Roll back onto roller with feet flat on floor. Place arms alongside roller. Raise one arm overhead. Lower arm to floor alongside roller. Repeat with opposite side.

HOLD: _____ second(s).   **REPEAT:** _____ time(s).   **FREQUENCY:** _____ x/day.

SPECIAL PROTOCOLS/NOTES: _____

_____

_____

PATIENT NAME:_____ DATE: _____

THERAPIST NAME: _____

Supine Unilateral Knee Lift

PURPOSE: To strengthen abdominal, back, and leg muscles.

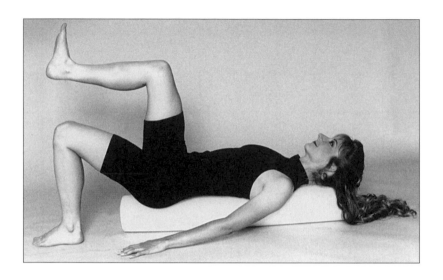

INSTRUCTION: Lie on side with knees bent. Roll back onto roller with feet flat on floor. Place arms alongside roller. Raise one knee toward chest. Maintain a 90-degree angle between knee and hip. Lower leg to floor. Repeat with opposite side.

HOLD: _____ second(s).   **REPEAT:** _____ time(s).   **FREQUENCY:** _____ x/day.

SPECIAL PROTOCOLS/NOTES: _____

_____

_____

PATIENT NAME:_____ DATE: _____

THERAPIST NAME: _____

Supine Spine Stabilization 90/90

PURPOSE: To strengthen abdominal, back, and leg muscles.

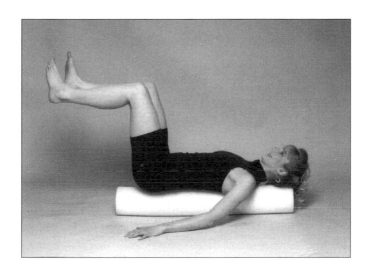

INSTRUCTION: Lie on side with knees bent. Roll back onto roller with feet off floor. Place arms alongside roller. Raise one knee, then second knee toward chest. Maintain a 90-degree angle between knees and hips.

HOLD: _____ second(s).   **REPEAT:** _____ time(s).   **FREQUENCY:** _____ x/day.

SPECIAL PROTOCOLS/NOTES: _____
_____
_____

PATIENT NAME:_____ DATE: _____
THERAPIST NAME: _____

Supine Spine Stabilization 90/90 with Shoulder Flexion

PURPOSE:　To strengthen abdominal, arm, back, neck, and leg muscles.

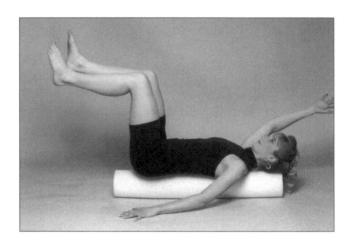

INSTRUCTION:　Lie on side with knees bent. Roll back onto roller with feet off floor. Place arms alongside roller. Raise one knee, then second knee toward chest. Maintain a 90-degree angle between knees and hips. Raise one arm overhead. Hold: _____ second(s). Lower arm to floor. Repeat with opposite arm.

REPEAT: _____ time(s). 　　　　　　**FREQUENCY:** _____ x/day.

SPECIAL PROTOCOLS/NOTES: _____

_____

_____

VARIATION:　Repeat exercise as above; however, lower both arms and legs between each exercise repetition. Relax. Repeat exercise sequence.

PATIENT NAME:_____ DATE: _____

THERAPIST NAME: _____

Supine Double Roller Shoulder Flexion

PURPOSE: To strengthen arm and neck muscles.

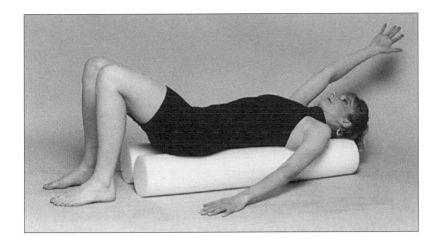

INSTRUCTION: Lie on back with knees bent. Roll back onto one roller. Place second roller parallel to first under back. Each roller should be on either side of back. Raise one arm overhead and lower. Repeat with opposite arm.

HOLD: _____ second(s).   **REPEAT:** _____ time(s).   **FREQUENCY:** _____ x/day.

SPECIAL PROTOCOLS/NOTES: _____

_____

_____

PATIENT NAME:_____ DATE: _____

THERAPIST NAME: _____

Supine Double Roller Knee Lift

PURPOSE: To strengthen abdominal, back, and leg muscles.

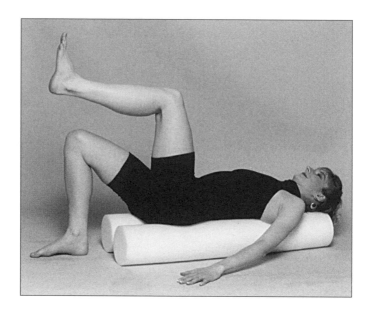

INSTRUCTION: Lie on side with knees bent. Roll back onto one roller. Place second roller parallel to first under back. Each roller should be on either side of spine. Raise one knee. Repeat with opposite knee.

HOLD: _____ second(s).   **REPEAT:** _____ time(s).   **FREQUENCY:** _____ x/day.

SPECIAL PROTOCOLS/NOTES: _____

_____

_____

PATIENT NAME:_____ DATE: _____

THERAPIST NAME: _____

Supine Double Roller Shoulder Flexion and Knee Lift

PURPOSE:　To strengthen abdominal, arm, back, leg, and neck muscles.

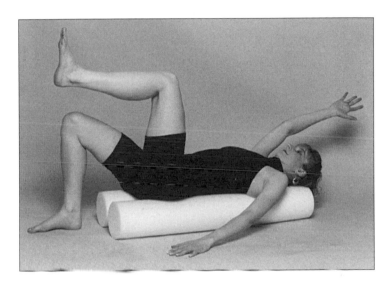

INSTRUCTION:　Lie on back with knees bent. Roll back onto one roller. Place second roller under back parallel to first. Each roller should be on either side of back. Raise one arm overhead while lifting opposite knee. Repeat with opposite side.

HOLD: _____ second(s).　**REPEAT:** _____ time(s).　**FREQUENCY:** _____ x/day.

SPECIAL PROTOCOLS/NOTES: _____

_____

_____

PATIENT NAME:_____ DATE: _____

THERAPIST NAME: _____

Supine Hip Extension

PURPOSE: To strengthen low back, buttock, leg, and ankle muscles.

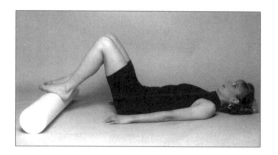

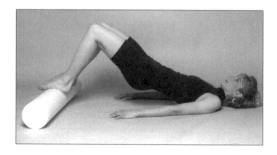

INSTRUCTION: Lie on back. Bend knees and place feet on roller. Lift hips off floor. Lower hips to floor.

HOLD: _____ second(s).   **REPEAT:** _____ time(s).   **FREQUENCY:** _____ x/day.

SPECIAL PROTOCOLS/NOTES: _____

_____

_____

PATIENT NAME:_____ DATE: _____

THERAPIST NAME: _____

Supine Hip Extension with Resistive Band Around Knees

PURPOSE: To strengthen low back, buttock, leg, and ankle muscles.

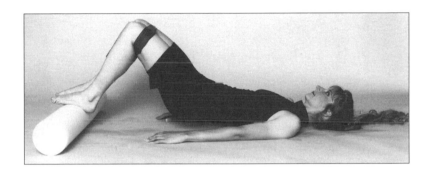

INSTRUCTION: Lie on back. Bend knees and place feet on roller. Wrap resistive band around knees and tie in knot. Lift hips off floor. Lower hips to floor.

HOLD: ____ second(s).   **REPEAT:** ____ time(s).   **FREQUENCY:** ____ x/day.

SPECIAL PROTOCOLS/NOTES: _____

_____

_____

PATIENT NAME:_____ DATE: _____

THERAPIST NAME: _____

Supine Hip Extension
with Feet on Ball

PURPOSE: To strengthen arm, back of leg, and buttock muscles. To improve balance reactions.

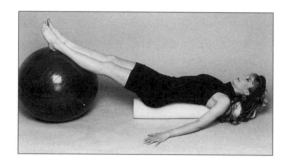

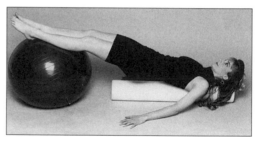

INSTRUCTION: Lie on side with knees bent. Roll back onto roller. Place ball under calves. Lift hips off roller.

HOLD: _____ second(s).   **REPEAT:** _____ time(s).   **FREQUENCY:** _____ x/day.

SPECIAL PROTOCOLS/NOTES: _____

_____

_____

PATIENT NAME:_____ DATE: _____

THERAPIST NAME: _____

Supine Hip Extension
with Heel Raise

PURPOSE: To strengthen ankle, buttock, leg, and low back muscles.

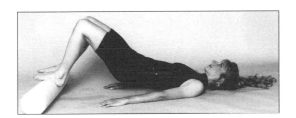

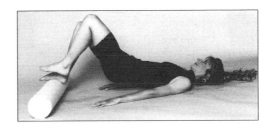

INSTRUCTION: Lie on back. Bend knees and place feet on roller. Lift hips off floor and raise right heel three inches off roller. Maintain neutral spine position. Return to starting position. Repeat with opposite side.

HOLD: ＿＿ second(s).　**REPEAT:** ＿＿ time(s).　**FREQUENCY:** ＿＿ x/day.

SPECIAL PROTOCOLS/NOTES: ＿＿＿＿＿＿＿＿＿＿＿＿＿＿＿＿＿＿＿
＿＿＿＿＿＿＿＿＿＿＿＿＿＿＿＿＿＿＿＿＿＿＿＿＿＿＿＿＿＿＿＿＿
＿＿＿＿＿＿＿＿＿＿＿＿＿＿＿＿＿＿＿＿＿＿＿＿＿＿＿＿＿＿＿＿＿

PATIENT NAME:＿＿＿＿＿＿＿＿＿＿＿＿＿＿＿＿＿ DATE: ＿＿＿＿＿＿

THERAPIST NAME: ＿＿＿＿＿＿＿＿＿＿＿＿＿＿＿＿＿＿＿＿＿

Supine Hip Extension with Knee Lift

PURPOSE: To strengthen ankle, buttock, leg, and low back muscles.

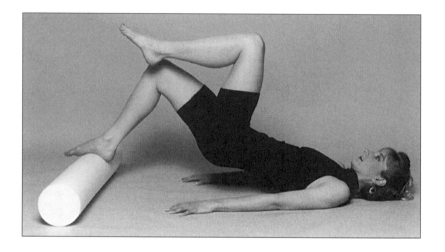

INSTRUCTION: Lie on back. Bend knees and place feet on roller. Lift hips off floor and raise one knee toward chest. Maintain neutral spine position. Return to starting position. Repeat with opposite side.

HOLD: _____ second(s).　**REPEAT:** _____ time(s).　**FREQUENCY:** _____ x/day.

SPECIAL PROTOCOLS/NOTES: _____

_____

_____

PATIENT NAME:_____ DATE: _____

THERAPIST NAME: _____

Supine Hip Extension with Knee Lift and Contralateral Shoulder Flexion

PURPOSE: To strengthen ankle, arm, buttock, leg, and low back muscles.

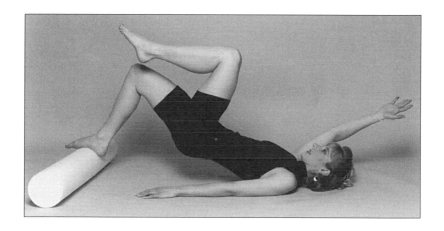

INSTRUCTION: Lie on back. Bend knees and place feet on roller. Lift hips off floor. Raise one knee toward chest and extend opposite arm overhead. Repeat with opposite arm and leg.

HOLD: _____ second(s).   **REPEAT:** _____ time(s).   **FREQUENCY:** _____ x/day.

SPECIAL PROTOCOLS/NOTES: _____
_____
_____

VARIATION: Repeat exercise as above; however, raise one knee toward chest and same side arm overhead. Repeat with opposite arm and leg.

PATIENT NAME:_____ DATE: _____

THERAPIST NAME: _____

Supine Isometric Hand Press

PURPOSE: To strengthen arm, hand, and forearm muscles.

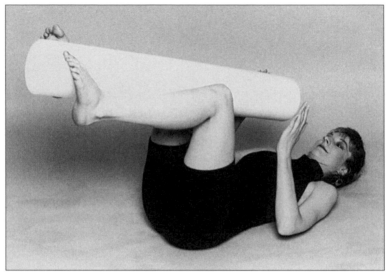

INSTRUCTION: Lie on back with knees bent. Raise both knees toward chest one at a time. Place roller between feet, knees, and hands. Press left hand into side of roller. Hold for _____ second(s). Repeat with right hand. Hold: _____ second(s).

REPEAT: _____ time(s).   **FREQUENCY:** _____ x/day.

SPECIAL PROTOCOLS/NOTES: _____
_____
_____

PATIENT NAME:_____ DATE: _____

THERAPIST NAME: _____

Supine Isometric Foot Press

PURPOSE: To strengthen inner thigh and leg muscles.

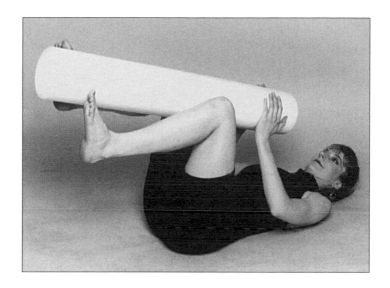

INSTRUCTION: Lie on back with knees bent. Raise both knees toward chest one at a time. Place roller between feet, knees, and hands. Press left foot into side of roller. Hold for _____ second(s). Repeat with right foot. Hold: _____ second(s).

REPEAT: _____ time(s).   **FREQUENCY:** _____ x/day.

SPECIAL PROTOCOLS/NOTES: _____
_____
_____

PATIENT NAME:_____ DATE: _____

THERAPIST NAME: _____

Supine Hip Internal and External Rotation with Small Ball

PURPOSE: To increase range of motion and strength in hips.

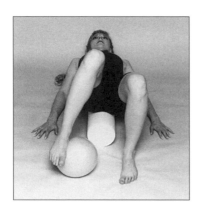

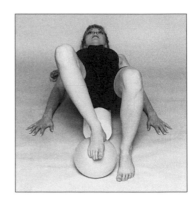

INSTRUCTION: Lie on side with knees bent. Roll back onto roller. Place hands at sides of body. Place ball under one foot. Gently roll ball away from opposite foot then gently roll ball toward opposite foot. Repeat with opposite side.

HOLD: ____ second(s).   **REPEAT:** ____ time(s).   **FREQUENCY:** ____ x/day.

SPECIAL PROTOCOLS/NOTES: _____

_____

_____

VARIATION: Lie on roller as above with hands at sides of body. Place ball under one foot. Lift hips off roller. Gently roll ball away from opposite foot then gently roll ball toward opposite foot. Repeat with opposite side.

PATIENT NAME:_____ DATE: _____

THERAPIST NAME: _____

Supine Straight Leg Raise
with Small Ball

PURPOSE: To strengthen abdominal, arm, back, buttock, and leg muscles.

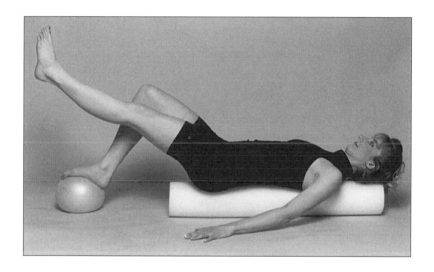

INSTRUCTION: Lie on side with knees bent. Roll back onto roller. Place small ball under right foot. Straighten left leg. Raise left leg. Repeat with opposite side.

HOLD: _____ second(s).   **REPEAT:** _____ time(s).   **FREQUENCY:** _____ x/day.

SPECIAL PROTOCOLS/NOTES: _____

_____

_____

VARIATION: Lie on side with knees bent. Roll back onto roller. Place small ball under right foot. Straighten left leg. Raise right arm overhead while raising left leg. Repeat with opposite side.

PATIENT NAME:_____ DATE: _____

THERAPIST NAME: _____

Supine Resistive Band Knee Extension

PURPOSE: To strengthen leg muscles.

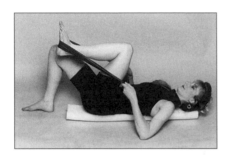

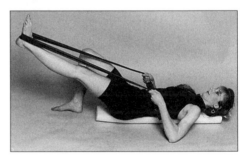

INSTRUCTION: Lie on side with knees bent. Roll back onto roller. Wrap ends of resistive band around each hand. Bend left knee toward chest. Place resistive band around arch of one foot. Extend that leg. Repeat with opposite leg.

HOLD: _____ second(s).　**REPEAT:** _____ time(s).　**FREQUENCY:** _____ x/day.

SPECIAL PROTOCOLS/NOTES: _____

_____

_____

PATIENT NAME:_____ DATE: _____

THERAPIST NAME: _____

Supine Hip Hiker
Quadratus Lumborum Exercise

PURPOSE: To strengthen hip and low back muscles.

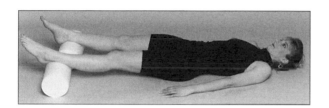

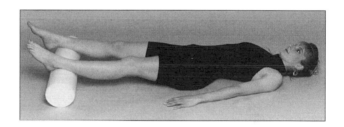

INSTRUCTION: Lie on back and place one small roller beneath each ankle. Straighten legs. Hike one hip toward shoulder. Repeat with opposite hip. Rollers should move independently of each other.

HOLD: _____ second(s). **REPEAT:** _____ time(s). **FREQUENCY:** _____ x/day.

SPECIAL PROTOCOLS/NOTES: Do not lift hips off floor. _____

_____

_____

PATIENT NAME:_____ DATE: _____

THERAPIST NAME: _____

CHAPTER NINE

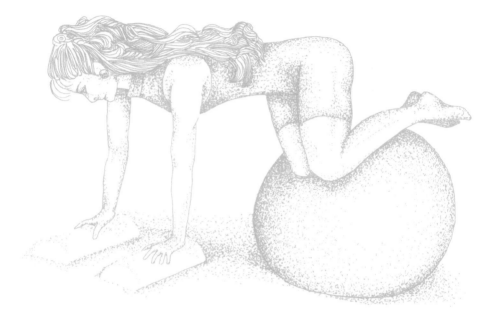

Sidelying and Prone Exercises

Sidelying and Prone Exercises

Sidelying Protraction/Retraction

PURPOSE: To increase range of motion in and strengthen shoulder muscles.

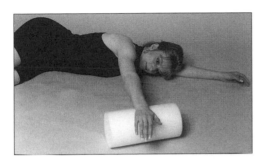

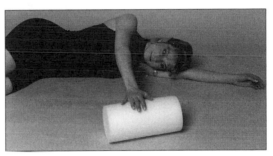

INSTRUCTION: Lie on side with knees bent. Extend one arm out away from body. Place small roller under that hand. Gently push roller out with shoulder. Repeat with opposite side.

HOLD: _____ second(s).   **REPEAT:** _____ time(s).   **FREQUENCY:** _____ x/day.

SPECIAL PROTOCOLS/NOTES: Do not bend elbow during exercise.
_____
_____

PATIENT NAME:_____ DATE: _____

THERAPIST NAME: _____

Sidelying Hip Extension

PURPOSE: To increase range of motion in and strengthen hip muscles.

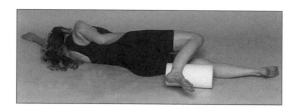

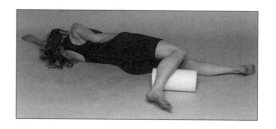

INSTRUCTION: Lie on side. Bend top knee and place foot on roller. Extend that leg out behind body. Repeat with opposite side.

HOLD: _____ second(s).   **REPEAT:** _____ time(s).   **FREQUENCY:** _____ x/day.

SPECIAL PROTOCOLS/NOTES: _____

_____

_____

PATIENT NAME:_____ DATE: _____

THERAPIST NAME: _____

Sidelying Hip Flexion

PURPOSE: To increase range of motion in and strengthen hip muscles.

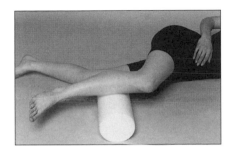

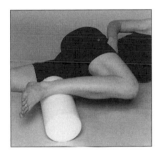

INSTRUCTION: Lie on side with bottom knee bent. Place top leg on small roller. Flex that knee toward chest. Repeat with opposite side.

HOLD: ____ second(s).   **REPEAT:** ____ time(s).   **FREQUENCY:** ____ x/day.

SPECIAL PROTOCOLS/NOTES: _____

_____

_____

_____

PATIENT NAME:_____ DATE: _____

THERAPIST NAME: _____

Prone Neutral Position

PURPOSE: To strengthen muscles in an optimal position to avoid injury.

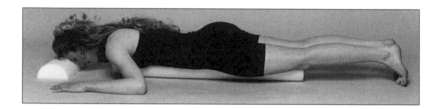

INSTRUCTION: Lie face down vertically on half roller with flat side up. Place small half roller under forehead. Place arms out at 70 degrees from body with elbows bent. Maintain natural curve in neck.

HOLD: _____ second(s).   **REPEAT:** _____ time(s).   **FREQUENCY:** _____ x/day.

SPECIAL PROTOCOLS/NOTES: <u>Do not flex or extend neck.</u>

_____

_____

PATIENT NAME:_____ DATE: _____

THERAPIST NAME: _____

Prone Balance

PURPOSE: To strengthen arm, back, and neck muscles. To improve balance reactions.

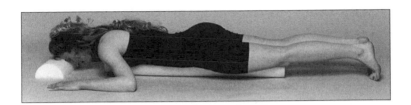

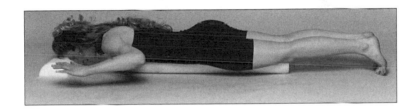

INSTRUCTION: Lie face down vertically on half roller with flat side up. Place small half roller under forehead. Place arms out at 70 degrees from body with elbows bent. Raise arms off floor.

HOLD: _____ second(s). **REPEAT:** _____ time(s). **FREQUENCY:** _____ x/day.

SPECIAL PROTOCOLS/NOTES: _____

_____

_____

VARIATION: a) Follow directions as above. Place arms out at 90 degrees with elbows bent. Raise arms off floor.
b) Follow directions as above. Raise arms overhead and turn thumbs toward ceiling. Raise one arm off floor. Lower arm to floor. Raise opposite arm off floor.

PATIENT NAME:_____ DATE: _____
THERAPIST NAME: _____

Prone Balance with Knee Flexion

PURPOSE: To strengthen arm, back, and neck muscles. To improve balance reactions.

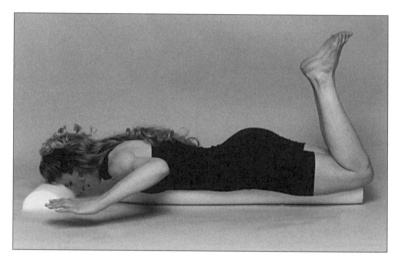

INSTRUCTION: Lie face down vertically on half roller with flat side up. Place small ball under forehead. Bend knees. Place arms out at 70 degrees from body with elbows bent. Raise arms off floor.

HOLD: _____ second(s).   **REPEAT:** _____ time(s).   **FREQUENCY:** _____ x/day.

SPECIAL PROTOCOLS/NOTES: _____

_____

_____

VARIATIONS: a) Follow directions as above. Place arms out at 90 degrees with elbows bent. Raise arms off floor.
b) Follow directions as above. Raise arms overhead and turn thumbs toward ceiling. Raise one arm off floor. Lower arm to floor. Repeat with opposite arm.

PATIENT NAME:_____ DATE: _____

THERAPIST NAME: _____

Prone Shoulder Flexion and Extension

PURPOSE: To increase shoulder range of motion. To strengthen arm and shoulder muscles.

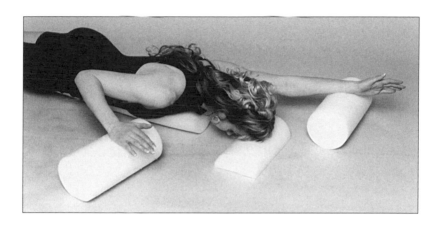

INSTRUCTION: Lie face down vertically on half roller with flat side up. Place small half roller under forehead with flat side down. Bend both elbows and place small rollers under each hand. Straighten left arm rotating thumb toward ceiling. Repeat with opposite side. Alternate bending and straightening arms in a gentle rhythmic pattern.

HOLD: _____ second(s). **REPEAT:** _____ time(s). **FREQUENCY:** _____ x/day.

SPECIAL PROTOCOLS/NOTES: _____
_____
_____

PATIENT NAME:_____ DATE: _____

THERAPIST NAME: _____

Prone Mid-Scapular Exercise

PURPOSE: To strengthen shoulder and mid back muscles.

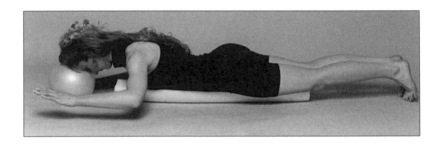

INSTRUCTION: Lie face down vertically on half roller with flat side up. Place small ball under forehead. Place arms out at 90 degrees from body with elbows bent. Gently move right shoulder blade toward floor and into spine. Raise one arm off floor. Repeat with opposite arm.

HOLD: _____ second(s).   **REPEAT:** _____ time(s).   **FREQUENCY:** _____ x/day.

SPECIAL PROTOCOLS/NOTES: Do not elevate shoulders toward ears during exercise.

PATIENT NAME:_____ DATE: _____

THERAPIST NAME: _____

Prone B.O.I.N.G.
Mid-Scapular Exercise

PURPOSE: To strengthen mid back and shoulder muscles.

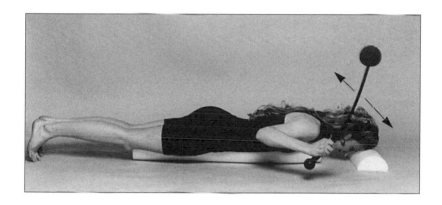

INSTRUCTION: Lie face down vertically on half roller with flat side up. Place small half roller under forehead. Place B.O.I.N.G. in one hand parallel to body. Move arms out away from body with elbows bent. Gently oscillate B.O.I.N.G. up and down. Repeat with opposite side.

HOLD: _____ second(s).   **REPEAT:** _____ time(s).   **FREQUENCY:** _____ x/day.

SPECIAL PROTOCOLS/NOTES: Do not tighten neck muscles while doing exercise.

VARIATION: Place one B.O.I.N.G. in each hand and follow directions as above.

PATIENT NAME:_____ DATE: _____

THERAPIST NAME: _____

Prone Bilateral Shoulder Flexion

PURPOSE: To strengthen arm, neck, shoulder, and upper and mid back muscles.

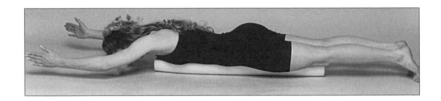

INSTRUCTION: Lie face down vertically on half roller with flat side up. Place small half roller under forehead with flat side down. Raise arms overhead. Rotate thumbs toward ceiling. Lift arms off floor. Lower arms to floor.

HOLD: _____ second(s).   **REPEAT:** _____ time(s).   **FREQUENCY:** _____ x/day.

SPECIAL PROTOCOLS/NOTES: Keep shoulders relaxed while lifting arms off floor.

VARIATION: Do exercise as above; however, lift one arm off floor at a time. Return to starting position. Lift opposite arm off floor.

PATIENT NAME:_____ DATE: _____

THERAPIST NAME: _____

Prone Tuck with Ball

PURPOSE: To strengthen abdominal, arm, and neck muscles. To increase range of motion in back.

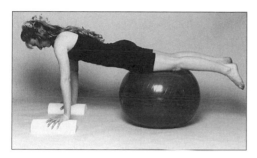

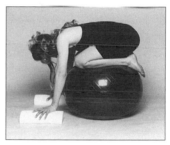

INSTRUCTION: Lie face down with abdomen on ball. Walk arms out until thighs are on ball. Place a half roller under each hand with flat sides down. Bring knees to chest until body is in a tuck position. Return to starting position.

HOLD: _____ second(s).   **REPEAT:** _____ time(s)   **FREQUENCY:**   x/day.

SPECIAL PROTOCOLS/NOTES: _____

_____

_____

PATIENT NAME:_____ DATE: _____

THERAPIST NAME: _____

Prone Skier

PURPOSE: To strengthen abdominal, arm, back, and neck muscles. To improve range of motion in back and hips.

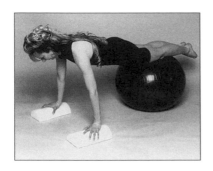

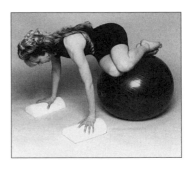

INSTRUCTION: Lie face down with abdomen on ball. Walk arms out until thighs are on ball. Place a half roller under each hand with flat sides down. Bend knees so right outer ankle is touching ball. Draw legs up to chest on left side. Repeat with opposite side.

HOLD: _____ second(s).   **REPEAT:** _____ time(s).   **FREQUENCY:** _____ x/day.

SPECIAL PROTOCOLS/NOTES: _____
_____
_____

PATIENT NAME:_____ DATE: _____
THERAPIST NAME: _____

Prone Tuck

PURPOSE: To increase range of motion in back and knees. To strengthen abdominal, arm, back, and neck muscles.

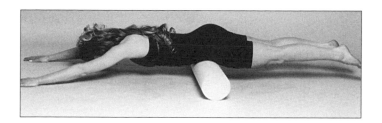

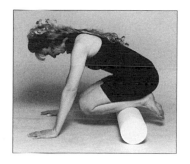

INSTRUCTION: Lie face down with abdomen over full roller placed horizontal on floor. Extend arms and legs. Lift both feet off floor. Pull knees up to chest until body is in a tuck position with hands flat on floor.

HOLD: _____ second(s).   **REPEAT:** _____ time(s).   **FREQUENCY:** _____ x/day.

SPECIAL PROTOCOLS/NOTES: _____

_____

_____

PATIENT NAME:_____ DATE: _____

THERAPIST NAME: _____

Prone Abdominal Crunch

PURPOSE: To strengthen arm and abdominal muscles.

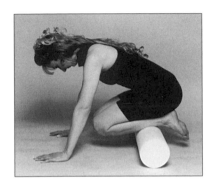

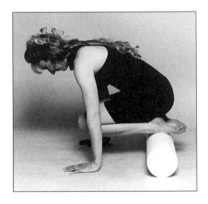

INSTRUCTION: Kneel. Place roller under both knees. Lean forward so hands touch floor with palms flat. Draw knees up toward chest.

HOLD: _____ second(s).   **REPEAT:** _____ time(s).   **FREQUENCY:** _____ x/day.

SPECIAL PROTOCOLS/NOTES: _____

_____

_____

PATIENT NAME:_____   DATE: _____

THERAPIST NAME: _____

Prone Push-Up I

PURPOSE: To strengthen muscles on front side of arm.

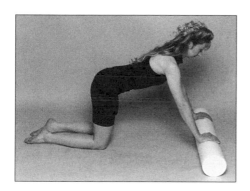

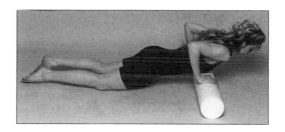

INSTRUCTION: Kneel. Place roller on floor horizontal in front of body. Lean forward so arms are extended out straight, hands are on top of roller, and body is in a modified push-up position. Slowly lower body down toward roller. Return to modified push-up position.

HOLD: _____ second(s).   **REPEAT:** _____ time(s).   **FREQUENCY:** _____ x/day.

SPECIAL PROTOCOLS/NOTES: Do not let stomach sag. _____

_____

_____

PATIENT NAME:_____ DATE: _____

THERAPIST NAME: _____

Prone Push-Up II

PURPOSE: To strengthen muscles on front side of arm.

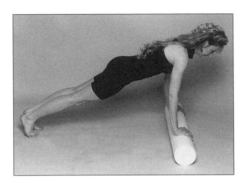

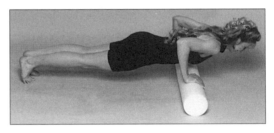

INSTRUCTION: Kneel. Place roller on floor horizontal in front of body. Lean forward so arms are extended out straight, hands are on top of roller, and body is in a modified push-up position. Slowly lower body down toward roller. Return to full push-up position.

HOLD: _____ second(s).   **REPEAT:** _____ time(s).   **FREQUENCY:** _____ x/day.

SPECIAL PROTOCOLS/NOTES: Do not let stomach sag._____

_____

_____

PATIENT NAME:_____ DATE: _____

THERAPIST NAME: _____

Prone Push-Up III

PURPOSE: To strengthen muscles on front side of arm.

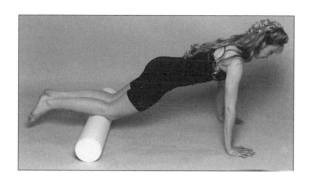

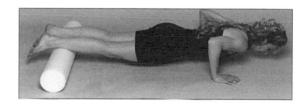

INSTRUCTION: Kneel. Place roller on floor horizontal in front of body under shins. Lean forward so hands are flat on floor and body is in a modified push-up position. Slowly lower body toward roller. Return to modified push-up position.

HOLD: _____ second(s).   **REPEAT:** _____ time(s).   **FREQUENCY:** _____ x/day.

SPECIAL PROTOCOLS/NOTES: Do not let stomach sag. _____

_____

_____

PATIENT NAME:_____ DATE: _____

THERAPIST NAME: _____

CHAPTER TEN

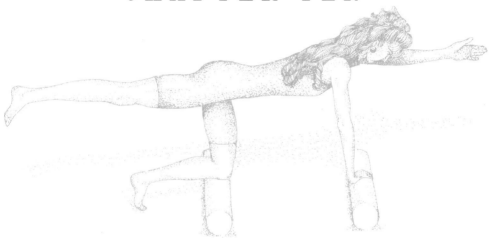

Case Studies

CASE STUDY 1

WRITTEN BY: Brian E. Hauswirth, P.T., C.F.P. (Certified
Feldenkrais Practitioner)
Foam Roller Instructor and Owner of
Integrating Function Physical Therapy,
Larkspur, CA.

DIAGNOSIS: Right hip tendonitis

HISTORY:

A thirty-one year old female with complaint of right lateral
hip pain when running. Symptoms began one year prior to
examination with competitive soccer and exacerbated and
remitted in relation to activity level.

Initially the patient complained of pain at the right hip and
inability to exercise and lie on the right side. She denied
parathesia, bowel/bladder disturbance, numbness/tingling, etc.
She was unable to jog more than one hundred yards before
producing sharp lateral hip pain.

On physical examination, the patient exhibited a positive
Thomas test for the anterior hip/thigh tightness with pain and
limited range of minus fifteen degrees. Attempts to adduct the
femur increased pain to the right lateral leg to mid thigh and
right hip.

Palpatory exam revealed mild generalized tenderness and
irritability of the entire right hip, however most
dysfunction/tenderness was noted at the iliac crest and tensor
fascia lata muscle. In standing the right ilium was elevated.

Light touch sensory exam and manual muscle test (MMT) of
L2-S1 was unremarkable. Deep tendon reflexes were
symmetrical in the lower extremities.

Single leg stance on the right produced a positive
Tredelenberg response after 30 seconds with inability to stabilize

the pelvis (i.e., drops on the left) and reproduction of pain.

Single leg bridge on the right was positive for inability to stabilize the pelvis (i.e., drops on the left) and reproduction of pain; fifteen seconds.

Trunk flexion to the left limited fifteen percent versus the right by right lateral hip pain.

TREATMENT:
Home Exercise Program
Frequency: 2 times per day
1) Supine Shoulder Rolls

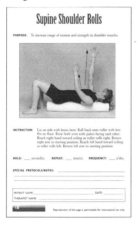

2) Iliotibial Band Massage

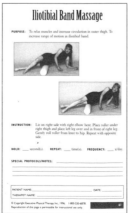

3) Hip Flexor Stretch

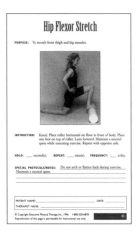

Hip Flexor Stretch

PURPOSE: To stretch front thigh and hip muscles.

INSTRUCTION: Kneel. Place roller horizontal on floor in front of body. Place one foot on top of roller. Lean forward. Maintain a neutral spine while executing exercise. Repeat with opposite side.

HOLD: ___ second(s).   **REPEAT:** ___ time(s).   **FREQUENCY:** ___ x/day.

SPECIAL PROTOCOLS/NOTES: Do not arch or flatten back during exercise. Maintain a neutral spine.

PATIENT NAME:_____ DATE:_____
THERAPIST NAME:_____

© Copyright Executive Physical Therapy, Inc., 1996.   1-800-330-6878
Reproduction of this page is permissible for instructional use only.

4) Standing Hip Hike

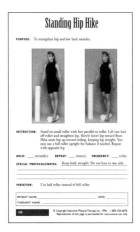

Standing Hip Hike

PURPOSE: To strengthen hip and low back muscles.

INSTRUCTION: Stand on small roller with feet parallel to roller. Lift one foot off roller and straighten leg. Slowly lower leg toward floor. Hike same hip up toward ceiling, keeping leg straight. You may use a full roller upright for balance if needed. Repeat with opposite leg.

HOLD: ___ second(s).   **REPEAT:** ___ time(s).   **FREQUENCY:** ___ x/day.

SPECIAL PROTOCOLS/NOTES: Keep body straight. Do not lean to one side.

VARIATION: Use half roller instead of full roller.

PATIENT NAME:_____ DATE:_____
THERAPIST NAME:_____

© Copyright Executive Physical Therapy, Inc., 1996.   1-800-330-6878
Reproduction of this page is permissible for instructional use only.

5) Supine Hip Extension

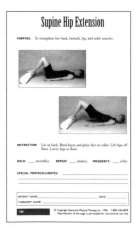

Supine Hip Extension

PURPOSE: To strengthen low back, buttock, leg, and ankle muscles.

INSTRUCTION: Lie on back. Bend knees and place feet on roller. Lift hips off floor. Lower hips to floor.

HOLD: ___ second(s).   **REPEAT:** ___ time(s).   **FREQUENCY:** ___ x/day.

SPECIAL PROTOCOLS/NOTES: _____

PATIENT NAME:_____ DATE:_____
THERAPIST NAME:_____

© Copyright Executive Physical Therapy, Inc., 1996.   1-800-330-6878
Reproduction of this page is permissible for instructional use only.

6) Supine Hip Extension with Knee Lift

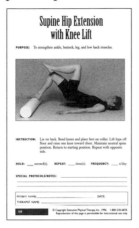

7) Supine Hip Extension with Resistive Band Around Knees

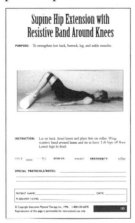

OUTCOME:

After two weeks of an independent home exercise program, performed twice a day, pain had decreased fifty percent, and the patient was able to jog for one mile.

After one month, the pain decreased eighty percent and patient was able to run 3–5 miles and restart soccer without pain. Palpation did not produce symptoms, Thomas test was negative, and stabilization improved to 2–3 minute tolerance on noted treatment positions.

CASE STUDY 2

WRITTEN BY: Caroline Corning Creager, P.T.
Foam Roller and Swiss Ball Instructor, Owner of
Executive Physical Therapy, Inc., Berthoud, CO.

DIAGNOSIS: Left acute inversion ankle sprain

HISTORY:

A thirty-six year old male engineer reported twisting his left
ankle while playing softball. He reports intermittent pain in his
left lateral malleolus region. Pain is nonexistent with non-
weight-bearing activities and is present with all weight-bearing
activities such as standing and walking (especially the toe-off
phase of gait). He stated he had twisted his left ankle at least
three times in the last fifteen years.

EVALUATION:

Minimal swelling noted inferior to left lateral malleolus.
Patient ambulates with antalgic gait on left side, a six-inch base
of support, and minimal toe off through gait cycle.

Tests for anterior talofibular ligament, posterior talofibular
ligament, and deltoid ligament were negative for instability.

Achilles tendon reflex was symmetrical bilaterally.

Patient demonstrated the following:

	left	right
MMT		
inversion	4/5 pain*	5/5
eversion	4/5	5/5
dorsiflexion	4+/5	5/5
plantarflexion	4/5	5–/5

---
*pain noted in left lateral malleolus region

ACTIVE RANGE OF MOTION IN SUPINE POSITION:

dorsiflexion	12	20
plantarflexion	32	42
inversion	08 pain*	18
eversion	05	05
hamstring	50	55
soleus	severe tightness; unable to flex knee for soleus stretch in standing	

BALANCE: < 5 seconds standing on full roller

---

*pain noted in left lateral malleolus region

TREATMENT:

FIRST DAY

Patient was instructed to do foam roller hamstring, gastrocnemius, and soleus stretches two times per day and was instructed in sitting active-assisted ankle plantarflexion and dorsiflexion range motion exercises to be done throughout day while sitting at his desk.

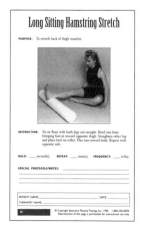

Long Sitting Hamstring Stretch

PURPOSE: To stretch back of thigh muscles.

INSTRUCTION: Sit on floor with both legs out straight. Bend one knee bringing foot in toward opposite thigh. Straighten other leg and place heel on roller. Flex toes toward body. Repeat with opposite side.

HOLD: ____ second(s).   REPEAT: ____ time(s).   FREQUENCY: ____ x/day.

SPECIAL PROTOCOLS/NOTES: _____

PATIENT NAME: _____ DATE: _____
THERAPIST NAME: _____

© Copyright Executive Physical Therapy, Inc., 1996.   1-800-530-6878.
Reproduction of this page is permissible for instructional use only.

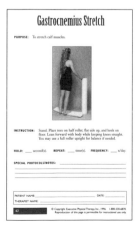

Gastrocnemius Stretch

PURPOSE: To stretch calf muscles.

INSTRUCTION: Stand. Place toes on half roller, flat side up, and heels on floor. Lean forward with body while keeping knees straight. You may use a full roller upright for balance if needed.

HOLD: ____ second(s).   REPEAT: ____ time(s).   FREQUENCY: ____ x/day.

SPECIAL PROTOCOLS/NOTES: _____

PATIENT NAME: _____ DATE: _____
THERAPIST NAME: _____

© Copyright Executive Physical Therapy, Inc., 1996.   1-800-530-6878.
Reproduction of this page is permissible for instructional use only.

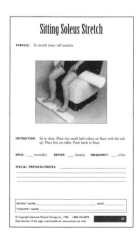

Sitting Soleus Stretch

PURPOSE: To stretch inner calf muscles.

INSTRUCTION: Sit in chair. Place two small half rollers on floor with flat side up. Place feet on roller. Push heels to floor.

HOLD: ____ second(s).   REPEAT: ____ time(s).   FREQUENCY: ____ x/day.

SPECIAL PROTOCOLS/NOTES: _____

PATIENT NAME: _____ DATE: _____
THERAPIST NAME: _____

© Copyright Executive Physical Therapy, Inc., 1996.   1-800-530-6878.
Reproduction of this page is permissible for instructional use only.

SECOND DAY

Patient reports that his ankle is feeling much better. Myofascial release and manual gastrocnemius, soleus, and anterior tibialis stretches performed on patient. He was instructed in standing foam roller balance exercise, mini knee bends, and side steps. Instructed patient in resistive band exercises for dorsiflexion, plantarflexion, eversion, and inversion. Reviewed exercise from first treatment.

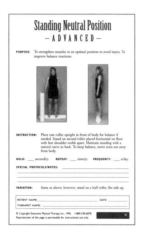

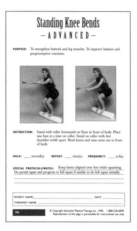

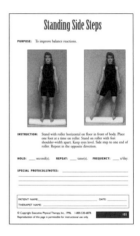

THIRD DAY

Ankle range of motion improving. Myofascial release performed to anterior foot. Range of motion exercises to left ankle in all planes. Foam roller exercises as previously.

FOURTH DAY

Patient reports no pain in ankle. Foam roller exercises as previously noted. Added side steps with knee bends with Swiss ball in hands. Swiss ball raised above head, above head side to side and proprioceptive neuromuscular facilitation (PNF) patterns.

FIFTH DAY

Range of motion and strength tests as noted below. Instructed in obstacle course on foam rollers with and without ball. Foam roller exercises as previously. Patient discharged from physical therapy, and was instructed to continue with his home exercise program.

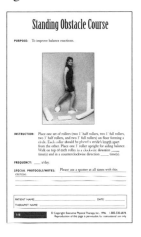

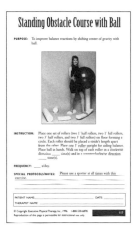

OUTCOME:

No complaints of pain in any weight-bearing position and no observable swelling noted. Pain-free gait, normal base of support (approximately 4 inches), and toe-off phase of gait was within normal limits.

MMTs presented grades bilaterally.

ACTIVE RANGE OF MOTION MEASUREMENTS:

dorsiflexion	20	20
plantarflexion	45	45
inversion	20	20
eversion	05	05
hamstring	65	65
soleus	within normal limits: able to do standing soleus stretch bending knee and keeping heel on floor.	

BALANCE: > 3 minutes standing on full foam roller

CASE STUDY 3

WRITTEN BY: Barbara J. Headley, M.S., P.T.
sEMG Instructor and Owner of Movement
Assessment, Research and Education Center,
Boulder, CO.

Therapists are choosing to use dynamic training more and more often. Swiss balls and foam rollers are being found often in orthopedic clinics, hospital outpatient clinics and even fitness centers. The concept of "dynamic stabilization" has caught on and almost every therapist can describe benefits of dynamic stabilization training. Others relate the use of such dynamic tools as foam rollers as a way of increasing the demand on muscles, making them work harder, and therefore providing an essential complement to strengthening. The component of postural control training may equal, or exceed, the benefits of foam rollers for increasing strength of certain muscle groups.

Perhaps the best way to understand the benefits of the dynamic foam roller exercises is to observe the differences in how individuals with chronic low back pain, for example, move as compared to individuals without pain. The particularly rigid gait of individuals with low back pain may be due to several factors. Muscle length changes may limit joint excursion, soft tissue adhesions may restrict tissue play,and pain alters muscle recruitment and changes motor strategies. Muscles may be inhibited, forcing compensatory muscle recruitment patterns. Central inhibition of muscles eventually affects motor strategies. As movement becomes restricted, the base of support narrows, limiting the ability to control balance when the center of gravity is challenged. Balancing reactions, defined as movements that attempt to maintain the center of gravity within the base of support, become limited, inefficient, and movement becomes more uncoordinated.

Many individuals with chronic pain or prolonged stiffness from injury have good strength. What they lack is the ability to coordinate their movement efficiently. The ability to develop the coordinated movement and balance necessary to provide a stable, dynamic base of support depends upon the relations of muscles at several joints such as in the relative timing and relative burst magnitudes and durations. Hence, the value of tools such as sEMG to evaluate muscle activity during dynamic exercise with the foam rollers, or any other type of exercise. The sEMG data is first a measure of how hard the muscle(s) are working. It is, therefore, a measure of strength during a given task. But no one muscle works in isolation. It must work with other muscles as a synergist symphony, not a chaotic riot. The sEMG data may have its greatest value in assessing the chaos, and assisting the therapist in facilitating a symphonic change in the muscle recruitment.

Movement is not measured by the strength of individual muscles; it is the ability to provide coordinated control of the constant loss of equilibrium. The task of postural adjustments is to correct equilibrium in the event of perturbation. Postural adjustments are accomplished by muscular activity within established strategies, already defined by central nervous system centers. Postural control in someone without pain, such as Caroline who produced these sEMG graphs, is more efficient and more coordinated than in someone with pain.

The sEMG data presented on several of the foam roller exercises in this chapter may give you some insight into how coordinated muscle activity should occur. Do not expect this type of activity from your patients. Muscle inhibition will be common in some; in others erratic high amplitude bursts of many muscles will deter coordinated movement. High amplitude, erratic sEMG patterns are seen in someone learning to perform a skilled movement for the first time. In many patients, the task of learning efficient movement again is as difficult as the first time. Monitoring some of the muscles so active in Caroline may demonstrate to you that muscle inhibition is part of your patient's movement dysfunction. Co-contraction of agonist and antagonist may also be a component of the movement dysfunction.

There is no normative data to show exactly how muscles should fire during these exercises. Amplitude may vary greatly within a group of individuals who are doing the exercises well. It is the relative muscle activity of one muscle to another within an individual that is most important.

Synopsis of microvolt readings for five foam roller exercises	Posterior Cervical	Lower Trapezius	Rectus Abdominus	Lumbar Paraspinal	Vastus Medialis Obliques	Hamstring	Anterior Tibialis	Gastro-cnemius
Standing Shoulder Flexion	50	600	125	30	50	80	160	140
Kneeling Balance	700	850	400	175	180	600	30	175
Supine 90/90	30	275	650	30	20	20	125	30
Supine Straight Leg Raise	850	250	900	30	30	80	200	180
Prone Shoulder Flexion/Extension	3500	20	20	20	20	10	50	20

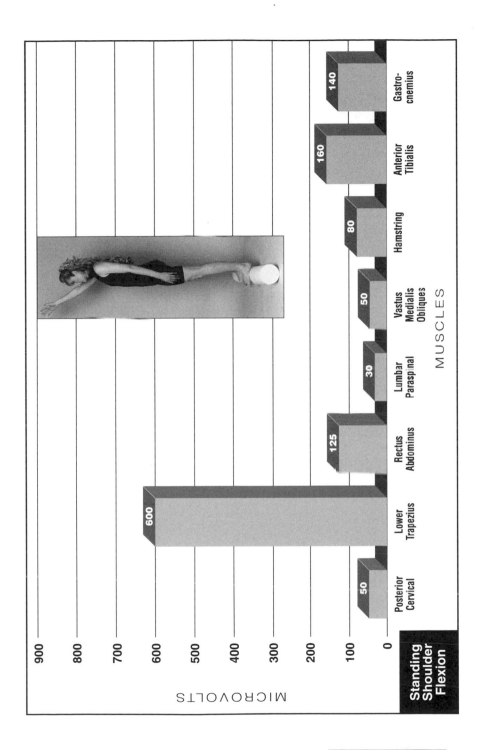

Standing Shoulder Flexion

MICROVOLTS

| | | Posterior Cervical | Lower Trapezius | Rectus Abdominus | Lumbar Paraspinal | Vastus Medialis Obliques | Hamstring | Anterior Tibialis | Gastro-cnemius |

Posterior Cervical: 50
Lower Trapezius: 600
Rectus Abdominus: 125
Lumbar Paraspinal: 30
Vastus Medialis Obliques: 50
Hamstring: 80
Anterior Tibialis: 160
Gastro-cnemius: 140

MUSCLES

229

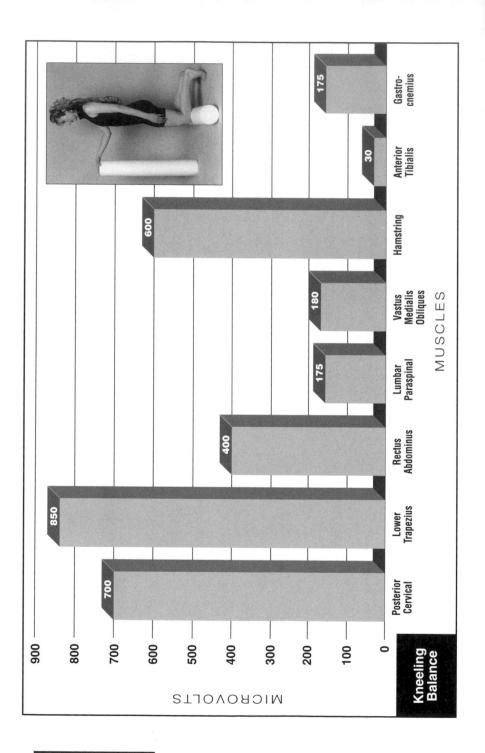

Kneeling
Balance

MUSCLES

MICROVOLTS

Posterior Cervical	700	
Lower Trapezius	850	
Rectus Abdominus	400	
Lumbar Paraspinal	175	
Vastus Medialis Obliques	180	
Hamstring	600	
Anterior Tibialis	30	
Gastro-cnemius	175	

230

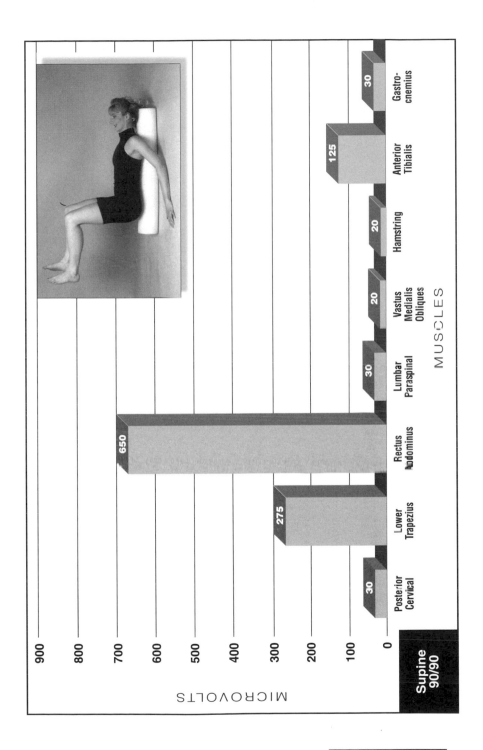

Supine 90/90

MICROVOLTS

Muscle	Value
Posterior Cervical	30
Lower Trapezius	275
Rectus Abdominus	650
Lumbar Paraspinal	30
Vastus Medialis Obliques	20
Hamstring	20
Anterior Tibialis	125
Gastro-cnemius	30

MUSCLES

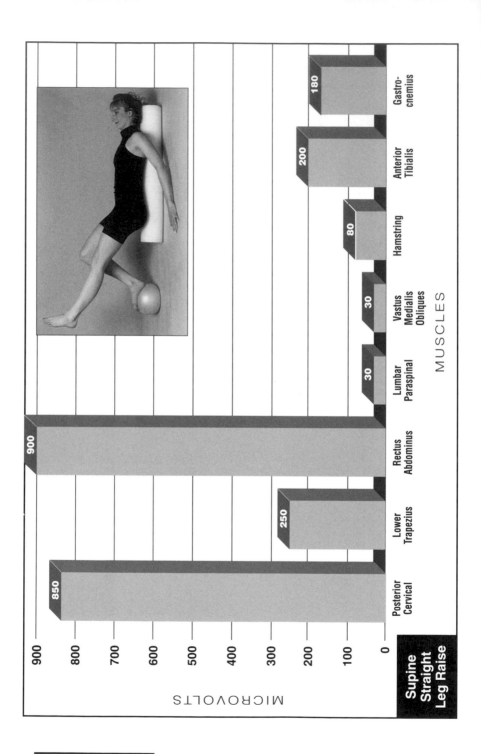

Supine Straight Leg Raise

MICROVOLTS

Muscle	Value
Posterior Cervical	850
Lower Trapezius	250
Rectus Abdominus	900
Lumbar Paraspinal	30
Vastus Medialis Obliques	30
Hamstring	80
Anterior Tibialis	200
Gastrocnemius	180

MUSCLES

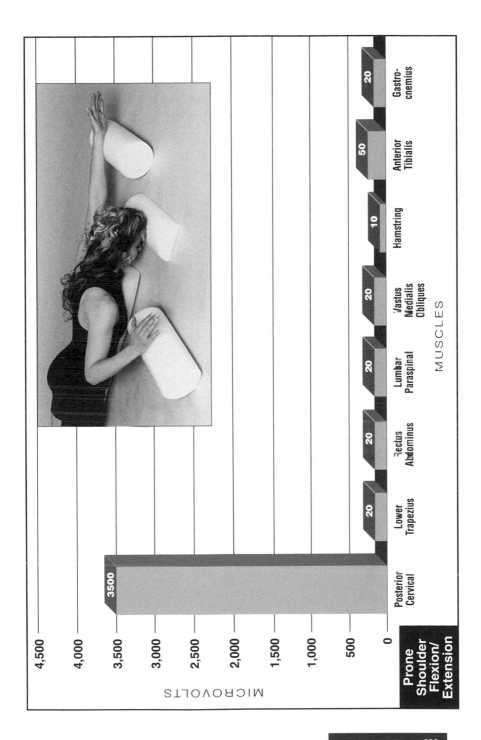

MICROVOLTS

4,500
4,000
3,500
3,000
2,500
2,000
1,500
1,000
500
0

Prone Shoulder Flexion/Extension

Posterior Cervical — 3500
Lower Trapezius — 20
Rectus Abdominus — 20
Lumbar Paraspinal — 20
Vastus Medialis Obliques — 20
Hamstring — 10
Anterior Tibialis — 50
Gastro-cnemius — 20

MUSCLES

References

Guyton, Arthur, 1991. *Textbook of Medical Physiology, Eighth Edition*. Philadelphia, PA: W.B. Saunders Company.

Johnson, Joan, 1995. *The Healing Art of Sports Massage*. Emmaus, PA: Rodale Press.

Hauswirth, Brian, and Kent Keyser. 1993. "Ethafoam Roller." *PT Magazine* (February): 93–94.

Maitland, G.D. 1986. *Vertebral Manipulation: Fifth Edition*. Butterworth & Co. Ltd.

Nail, Elsa. 1994. *Body and Soule: Soule roll integrated exercise program*. Tampa, FL.

Parker, Ilana. 1992. *Functional Exercise Program Seminar Workbook 1993*. San Francisco, CA.

Rocobado, Marianno. 1993. *Introduction to the Thoracic Region and the Rib Cage Workbook, 1996*. Tucson, AZ: IFORC.

Recommended Reading

 Creager, Caroline Corning. *Core Strength Training using Inflatable and Foam Rollers*, Berthoud, CO: Executive Physical Therapy Inc., 2006.

 Creager, Caroline Corning. *Bounce Back Into Shape After Baby*, Berthoud, CO: Executive Physical Therapy Inc., 2001.

 Creager, Caroline Corning. *The Airobic Ball™ Strengthening Workout*, Berthoud, CO: Executive Physical Therapy Inc., 1994.

 Creager, Caroline Corning. *The Airobic Ball™ Stretching Workout*, Berthoud, CO: Executive Physical Therapy Inc., 1995.

 Creager, Caroline Corning. *Therapeutic Exercises Using the Swiss Ball*, Berthoud, CO: Executive Physical Therapy Inc., 1994.

 Creager, Caroline Corning. *Therapeutic Exercises Using Resistive Bands*, Berthoud, CO: Executive Physical Therapy Inc., 1998.

Hosting and Open & Closed Chain Stabilization Course, Swiss Ball, or Foam Roller Courses

By Caroline Corning Creager, P.T.

If you are interested in hosting an open and closed chain course, swiss ball, or foam roller course, please call 1-800-530-6878 or 970-532-2533, or email: Caroline@CarolineCreager.com.

Visit our website at:
www.CarolineCreager.com

CAROLINE CREAGER'S
Carrying Strap
for
FOAM ROLLERS
& SWISS BALLS

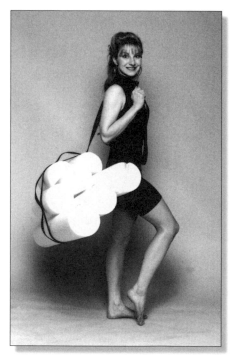

"I have found the easiest way to carry foam rollers or Swiss balls is by using a carrying strap! Also, try using the strap with stretching exercises on the ball or rollers."
Caroline Creager, P.T.

Ordering Information

To obtain more information about ordering exercise balls
and books please call the following distributors:

AUSTRALIA
Healthtrek: 0500 888843, www.healthtrek.net
OR
Star Systems: 02 6772 7433, www.starsystems.com.au

NEW ZEALAND
Network for Fitness Professionals: 09 479 8635
Email: info@netfitpro.co.nz

SOUTH AFRICA
Thera Med: 27 11 8046746
home.global.co.za/~dhtgo/

UNITED KINGDOM
Russell Medical:
01684 311 444
Email: enquiries@russellmedical.co.uk
OR
Physical Company Ltd: 01494 769 222
www.physicalcompany.co.uk

UNITED STATES & CANADA
Orthopedic Physical Therapy Products:
(800) 367-7393 or (763) 553-0452
www.optp.com

Visit our website at:
www.CarolineCreager.com

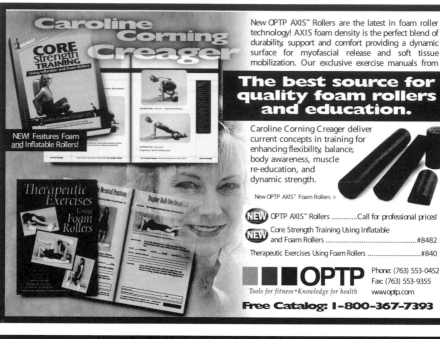
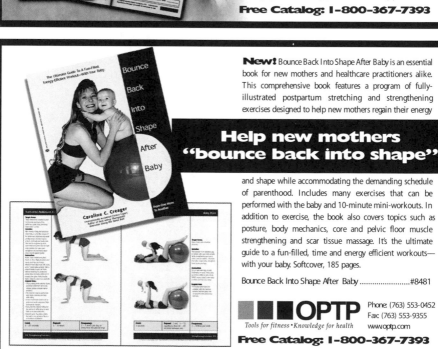

Index

abdominal muscles: exercises
to strengthen, 82, 98, 101,
102, 153, 154, 161, 164,
165, 168, 169, 171, 172,
173, 174, 175, 176, 177,
178, 179, 180, 182, 183,
193, 209, 210, 211, 212.
Airobic balls. *See* Swiss balls.
angina, 6.
ankle muscles: exercises to
increase range of motion
in, 126, 127; exercises to
strengthen, 109, 110, 111,
184, 185, 187, 188, 189;
stretching exercises, 58,
62, 63, 64.
ankle sprain: 15, 222-225;
exercises to strengthen, 71,
103, 105, 106, 116, 117;
stretching exercises, 58,
62, 63, 64.
anterior cruciate ligament, 2.
arm muscles: exercise to
increase range of motion
in, 155; exercises to
strengthen: 76, 77, 78, 79,
80, 81, 94, 95, 96, 97, 98,
101, 102, 112, 113, 114,
129, 130, 131, 136, 138,
152, 154, 155, 156, 160,
161, 164, 165, 168, 169,
171, 172, 177, 180, 181,
183, 186, 189, 190, 193,

203, 204, 205, 208, 209,
210, 211, 212, 213, 214,
215; stretching exercise,
46.

back muscles: exercises to
increase range of motion
in, 48, 49, 50, 52, 122, 123,
140, 141, 173, 209, 210,
211; exercises to
strengthen, 99, 101, 102,
108, 112, 113, 114, 124,
137, 138, 161, 165, 170,
172, 177, 178, 179, 180,
182, 183, 184, 185, 187,
188, 189, 193, 195, 203,
204, 206, 207, 208, 210,
211; stretching exercise,
51.

balance reactions: 2, 4; as
protocol for using foam
rollers, 6; exercises to
improve, 70, 71, 74, 75,
76, 77, 78, 79, 80, 81, 94,
95, 96, 97, 100, 103, 104,
105, 106, 112, 113, 114,
115, 116, 117, 143, 144,
145, 146, 160, 161, 186,
203, 204.
Barbis, John, 27.
B.O.I.N.G.s: principles and
concepts of, 19-20; used in

exercises with foam rollers,
94, 95, 96, 97, 98, 101,
102, 170, 172, 207.
breathing, 24-26, 28-30.
buttock muscles: exercise to
improve circulation, 54;
exercise to increase range
of motion in 54; exercises
to strengthen, 104, 105,
106, 107, 109, 110, 111,
137, 184, 185, 186, 187,
188, 189, 193; stretching
exercises, 55, 56.

calf muscles, stretching
exercises, 62, 63, 64.
cardiovascular distress, signs
of, 6.
carpal tunnel syndrome: 7-8;
exercises for treatment of,
42, 43, 44, 45, 211;
prevention of, 34, 37.
case studies: left ankle
inversion ankle sprain,
222-225; right hip
tendonitis 218-221; sEMG
data from foam roller
exercise, 226-233.
cerebrovascular accident: 16;
exercises for treatment of,
128, 195, 199, 200, 201.
cervical strain: 11; exercises
for treatment of, 72, 74,
80, 151, 208.
chest breathing, 28.
chest muscles: exercise to
strengthen, 156; stretching
exercise, 44.
computer fitness: 34-37; and

computer monitors, 34, 35;
and keyboards, 34, 37; and
lighting, 36; and seated
posture, 35-36, 37; and
special equipment, 36-37.
coordination, as protocol for
using foam rollers, 6.
Creager, Caroline Corning,
222-225.

degenerative joint disease,
aggravating with mobility
exercises, 6.
diaphragmatic breathing,
28-30.
diaphragmatic breathing
exercise, 30.
diaphragm muscle, role in
breathing, 24-25.
dizziness, 6.
Dyna-Brand®. *See* resistive
bands.
dynamic stabilization,
226-228.

endurance, as protocol for
using foam rollers, 6.
Ethafoam®, 2-3, 5.
exhaling, 24.
expiration, 25.
eye movement, exercises to
disassociate from neck
movement, 72, 73.
eye-hand coordination,
exercise to improve, 164.

Feldenkrais Method, the, 3.
Feldenkrais, Moshe, 3.
flushing, 6.

foam rollers: care and cleaning of, 5; contraindications for use of, 7; design of, 2-3; kneeling exercises using, 134, 142-146; patient compliance with, 2; precautions for use of, 6-7; principles and concepts of, 2-5; prone exercises using, 198, 202-215; protocol for use of, 6-7; quadriped exercises using, 134, 135-141; sidelying exercises using, 198, 199-201; sitting exercises using, 120, 121-131; sizes of, 3-4; standing exercises using, 68-69, 70-117; stretching exercises using, 40, 41-64; supine exercises using, 148-149, 150-195; treatment protocols with, 7-18; used to diversify exercise regimen, 2.

forearm muscles, exercises to strengthen, 94, 95, 96, 97, 190.

full foam rollers, use of, 4.

Greenburg, David, 19.

half foam rollers, use of, 4.

hand muscles, exercises to strengthen, 94, 95, 96, 97, 190.

Hauswirth, Brian, 2, 218-221.

head, exercises to disassociate from trunk, 74, 75.

Headley, Barbara J., 226-228.

hemiplegia, 16.

hip muscle: exercises to increase range of motion in, 141, 192, 200, 201, 210; exercises to strengthen, 108, 139, 174, 192, 195, 200, 201; stretching exercise, 53.

hip tendonitis, 218-221; exercises for treatment of, 53, 61, 108, 158, 184, 185, 188.

Hulme, Janet, 28, 29.

ilitibial band, exercise to increase range of motion in, 61; exercise to strengthen, 61.

inhaling, 24.

injury precautions, 6.

injury, exercises to help avoid, 70, 71, 121, 135, 142, 150, 202.

inner calf muscles, stretching exercises, 63, 64.

inner thigh muscles: exercise to improve circulation, 60; exercise to increase range of motion, 60; exercise to strengthen, 191.

inspiration, 25.

knees, exercises to increase range of motion in, 128, 211.

kneeling exercises, 134, 142-146.

lateral epicondylitis, 9;
exercises for treatment of,
42, 43, 46, 94, 211.
leg muscles, exercises to
strengthen, 101, 102, 104,
105, 106, 107, 109, 110,
111, 112, 113, 114, 124,
125, 128, 137, 138, 144,
145, 146, 153, 154, 161,
174, 178, 179, 180, 182,
183, 184, 185, 186, 187,
188, 189, 191, 193, 194.
light-headedness, 6.
low back muscles: exercises to
increase range of motion
in, 50, 122, 123, 141, 173;
exercises to strengthen,
108, 179, 184 185, 187,
188, 189, 195; stretching
exercise, 51.
low back pain, 12; exercises
to alleviate, 50, 51, 59,
179, 195; use of McKenzie
Lumbar Roll to alleviate,
35-36.
lower abdominal muscles,
exercises to strengthen,
175, 176.
lower oblique abdominal
muscles, exercise to
strengthen, 176.

McKenzie Lumbar Roll,
35-36.
mid back: exercises to
increase range of motion
in, 49, 140; exercises to
strengthen, 99, 170, 206,
207, 208.

motor loss, treatment of, 16.
See also cerebrovascular
accident.
motor planning, as protocol
for using foam rollers, 6.
multiple sclerosis, 17;
exercises for treatment of,
99, 107, 112, 175, 184.
muscle length, increasing, 41.
muscular fatigue, 6.
muskoskeletal disorders and
respiratory dysfunction,
27.
myofascial tissue, as protocol
for using foam rollers, 6.

Nail, Elsa, 2.
nausea, 6.
neck muscles, exercises to
strengthen, 124, 136, 138,
151, 152, 153, 154, 168,
169, 171, 180, 181, 183,
203, 204, 208, 209, 210,
211.
neural flexibility, as protocol
for using foam rollers, 6.
neutral spine position,
exercises to promote, 122,
123.
oblique abdominal muscles,
exercises to strengthen,
173, 174, 176.
office lighting, 36.
outer thigh muscles: exercise
to increase circulation, 61;
exercise to relax, 61.

pallor, 6.
Parker, Ilana, 2.